Hairdressing and Science:
A competence-based approach

Stephanie Henderson and Marion Phillips

STANLEY THORNES (Publishers) LTD

Originally published in 1988 by Hutchinson Education
Reprinted 1989

Reprinted again in 1989 by
Stanley Thornes (Publishers) Ltd
Old Station Drive
Leckhampton
CHELTENHAM GL53 0DN

British Library Cataloguing in Publication Data
Hairdressing and Science
1. Hairdressing
646.7'242

ISBN 0 7487 0286 5

Typeset in 11/14pt Palatino
Printed and bound in Great Britain at The Bath Press, Avon

CONTENTS

ABOUT THE AUTHORS

Stephanie Henderson LCG Cert.Ed
Past Senior Lecturer in Charge of Hairdressing School at Basingstoke Technical College, and Examiner for Advanced City and Guilds Ladies Hairdressing written paper, Practical Assessor for City and Guilds 300/1 Competence Certificate.

Marion Phillips B.Sc, C.Biol, MI Biol, Cert.Ed
A scientist with extensive lecturing experience including Hairdressing Science and Health studies.

ABOUT THE BOOK

This book contains all the necessary text for the City and Guilds 300/1 Hairdressing Certificate and the Hairdressing Training Board National Preferred scheme including background and supplementary science and design studies. It will also prove invaluable for anyone taking RIPHH Certificate in Salon Hygiene for Hairdressers, and The Guild of Hairdressers National Diploma for Hairdressers.

Each chapter relates to a 'hairdressing competence' in the practical aspects of hairdressing, and contains practice multiple choice questions.

If all else fails read the instructions!

By reading this book you will learn not only what will make you a good hairdresser and how to be successful, but also why things happen the way they do.

1

INDUSTRIAL STUDIES

Career Patterns

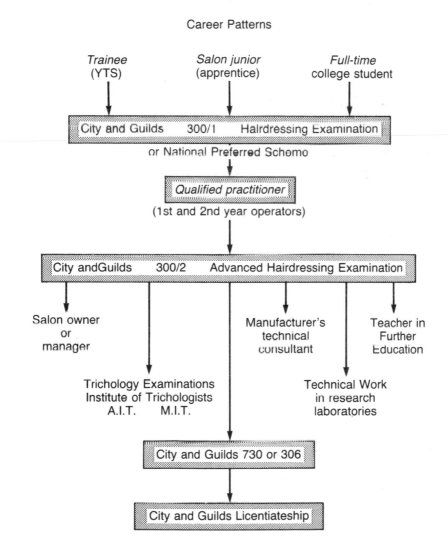

There are a variety of careers associated with the hairdressing industry. These two charts should give you an idea of how you can get into hairdressing and what you can do once you have qualified.

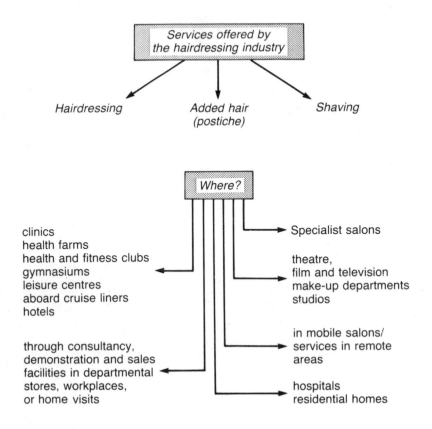

2

SAFETY, HEALTH AND HYGIENE PRACTICES

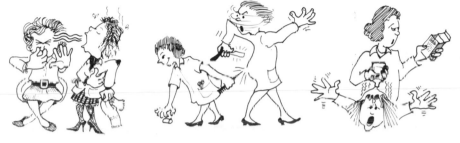

SAFETY IN THE SALON

Hairdressers must always work:

1 **Carefully** — Careless work could lead to hair loss, hair breakage, damage to the client's skin or eyes, or ruined clothes.

2 **Cleanly** — Tools and equipment must be clean and properly sterilized. What disease could the client catch from dirty equipment? What could you catch?

3 **Tidily** — Hairdressers cannot work quickly and efficiently if tools and equipment are muddled.

Protective clothing

No matter how careful hairdressers are, there is always the danger that chemicals such as permanent wave lotion, bleaches and hair colours may spill on to their clothes. Therefore, protective clothing is vital. Overalls, dye aprons and rubber gloves should always be worn when using hazardous chemicals.

The client's protection is equally important, not only when applying chemicals to the hair but for general cutting and styling too. Gowns, shoulder capes, towels, tissues and cotton wool strips should be used for the appropriate treatment.

Safe handling of tools

Many sharp and dangerous tools are used by hairdressers, such as scissors, open (cut-throat) razors, and pin-tail combs. Never keep any tools in your pockets or anywhere unsafe (e.g. on chairs, or protruding from trolleys). If anyone should trip over or fall they could cut, injure or stab themselves.

Safe handling of chemicals

Chemicals such as permanent wave lotion, bleaches, tints and hydrogen peroxide can burn the skin — so handle them with care! All manufacturers issue instructions, either on a leaflet (inside the box) or on the outside of the box. Always read the instructions carefully before starting any process.

Hazards in the salon

Carelessness in the salon is caused by lack of training, lack of supervision, insufficient experience, tiredness or even through drinking alcohol or drug-taking. Look carefully at the following table which shows what could happen.

Possible accident	Cause
Chemical burns (see Chapter 11)	Spilt permanent wave lotions. Spilt hydrogen peroxide. Incompatible chemicals (such as metallic dyes and hydrogen peroxide) used on hair, creating enough heat to burn the skin.
Physical burns (see page 9)	Electric tongs, hot brushes, hair dryers, accelerators or infra-red bulbs near the skin.

Possible accident	Cause
Scalds *(see page 9)*	Boiling water or steamers burning the skin.
Allergies *(see page 69)*	Permanent dyes used without a skin test which cause a reaction (contact dermatitis).
Cuts *(see page 9)*	Scissors, open razors or broken glass.
Infection *(see page 11 and 15)*	Little or no treatment of injuries. Inadequate sterilization of tools and equipment.
Falls *(see page 6)*	Slippery floors from water, oil, shampoo or grease spillages. Blocked passageways.
Electric shock *(see page 23)*	Water and electricity. Electrical appliances with poor insulation.
Poisoning	Drinking from incorrectly labelled bottles. Dangerous vapours from ammonia and dry cleaning fluids.
Fire *(see page 18)*	Hairdressing chemicals such as ethyl acetate (nail varnish remover) and hair lacquer are highly inflammable. Smoking.

Any accidents must be recorded in the accident register (see page 6).

Salon staff must work safely to protect themselves and their clients whilst in the salon. They must know all the possible dangers, how to protect themselves and their clients and how to prevent accidents.

SAFETY AND THE LAW

The following acts contain legal regulations which apply to the salon environment:

The Health and Safety at Work Act, 1974
The Factories Act, 1961
The Offices, Shops and Railway Premises Act, 1963

Employer's duties

Employers must provide the following:

1   A safe place of work, e.g. safe entrance and exit.
2   Safe, well-maintained equipment.
3   Safe systems and methods of work.
4   Protective clothing where applicable.
5   A safe working environment which incorporates the following:
  (a)   The maintenance of reasonable working temperatures — not less than 16°C (60.8°F) after the first hour (a thermometer to be provided).
  (b)   The maintenance of ventilation and humidity levels, fume and dust control.
  (c)   Suitable and sufficient lighting.
  (d)   The provision of adequate washing facilities. Sanitation — up to five employees of either sex, one toilet; over five employees one for each sex, over ten employees (and if the public have access) extra toilets must be provided.
  (e)   The provision of first aid facilities — a first aid box containing only first aid requisites must be readily accessible (see page 10).
  (f)   Safe methods of handling, storing and transporting goods and disposal of waste. Chemicals and dangerous materials, e.g. hydrogen peroxide, permanent wave lotion, bleaches and 'para' dyes, must be stored safely, and correctly labelled. Areas where chemicals are stored, dispensed and mixed together must be properly ventilated.
  (g)   The reporting of all accidents in the accident register, and the enforcing authority to be notified when the accident either causes the death of a person employed to work on the premises, or disables anyone for more than three days from doing their work. This law is also covered by the regulations in Safety Representatives and Safety Committees 1977, and Notifications of Accidents and General Occurences Regulations, 1980.
  (h)   Salon information, instruction training and supervision of employees must all be maintained.
  (i)   A safety policy regarding the Health and Safety at Work Act must be provided and be subject to regular review by both employers' and employees' representatives.

Employee's duties

Employees must take care of their own health and safety and that of anyone who may be affected by their work. This involves:

1 Having some knowledge of first aid.
2 Being aware of the potential for accidents and having the foresight to prevent them. Being able to locate the water stop-tap and the mains electricity cut off switch and gas tap.
3 Knowing how to telephone for an ambulance or for the fire service.
4 Understanding how to use the fire extinguisher.

Enforcement

Depending on the type of premises, enforcement of the law is carried out by local authorities (Environmental Health Officers) or Factory Inspectors.

The Health and Safety Executive has appointed inspectors who have power at any reasonable time to enter premises. They may issue either improvement or prohibition notices. Failure to comply with these is a criminal offence punishable by a fine or imprisonment.

Negligence

Negligence means the failure to use care. The law states that any task performed in the salon which may give rise to danger must be done competently.

Being aware of the law is not enough! Accidents can and do happen. **Who is responsible? What can be done about it?**

NEGLIGENCE toward the client This can involve damage to or loss of the client's clothes or belongings, e.g. jewellery (earrings, necklaces, rings, etc) or purses, handbags and shopping. Every hairdresser has a duty to take reasonable care of the client's safety and well-being, otherwise the client may claim compensation.

In all cases of injury or damage the manager must be called. The hairdresser must be sympathetic, but say nothing to the client which may suggest that they have accepted liability for the accident. Any first aid should be given at the order of the manager.

Full details of the incident including a written statement from the hairdresser who attended the client, must be sent to the Insurance Company immediately.

EMPLOYEE NEGLIGENCE Employees have a duty to work safely and responsibly. This includes honesty whilst dealing with money, and locking up the premises securely at night.

EMPLOYER NEGLIGENCE Employers have a duty to provide a safe system of working.

Insurance policies

Insurance policies may cover general insurance, public liability and employer's liability.

GENERAL INSURANCE This covers the following points:

1 **Structure** —	the building is covered for storm damage, explosions or floods from burst pipes.
2 **Fire** —	damage to structure and loss of profits during repair are also covered.
3 **Contents** —	as for the structure of the building, and for burglary.
4 **Loss of money** —	dishonesty of clients and employees.
5 **Fidelity** —	any financial loss due to fraud or theft by staff handling cash.

PUBLIC LIABILITY This is where the client claims as a result of damage or injuries received during treatment.

EMPLOYERS' LIABILITY This concerns accidents to employees in the course of their work, e.g. from faulty equipment, bodily injury or disease.

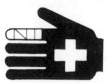

FIRST AID

First aid usually involves immediate treatment of minor accidental injuries, but may be necessary for more serious injuries before they are seen by a doctor. The aim is to prevent death or further damage to injured persons. If in any doubt about an injury, always seek medical advice from a doctor or nurse at a health clinic or the Casualty Department at a hospital.

It is not possible here to give full details of first aid treatments but some guidelines are given in the following table.

Injury	Treatment
Cut	Keep the wound clean to help stop infection. All open wounds or cuts should be covered. Do not allow blood or lesion to come into contact with other people or instruments (AIDS risk, see page 13 and 15).
Bruises	Apply a cold compress (e.g. ice or witch-hazel).
Burns and scalds	Hold affected area under running cold water tap or apply ice-pack (5-10 minutes). If the skin is broken or blistered, cover with a sterile dressing to help stop infection. Burns can be very serious, so seek medical advice unless the burn is very minor.
Fainting	Fainting is caused by insufficient blood supplied to the brain. Lowering the head and raising the feet will increase the blood supply to the brain.
Epileptic fit	The person may fall unconscious and limbs may jerk violently. Do not restrain movements but prevent damage to the person by removing nearby objects. The person will regain consciousness in a short time but may need to rest or sleep.
Accidents to the eye Chemicals in the eye	Wash the eye with running water (under the tap if possible or using an eye-wash cup). Continue applying water to the eye until medical assistance is available.
Foreign bodies in the eye	Try to remove the foreign bodies by washing out with water. Do not rub the eye.
Eye wounds	Do not attempt to treat these yourself. Always seeks medical advice.
Heart attack/cardiac arrest	The symptoms for this are a sudden crushing vice-like pain in the chest, breathlessness and a fast weakening pulse. Gently sit the patient down and seek immediate medical assistance. If the heart stops beating altogether begin resuscitation immediately.

Resuscitation techniques

You will need to get full details of these techniques from a qualified first aider or a First Aid manual. The main steps are:

1 Ensure an open airway.
2 Breathe for the casualty by inflating the lungs (artificial respiration).
3 Circulate the blood by compressing the chest.

Calling for assistance

If an accident happens you should call for assistance immediately by contacting the relevant emergency service: the ambulance, Police, Fire Brigade or the utilities, e.g. Gas or Electricity Boards.

999 CALLS — Fire, Police and Ambulance services   Dial 999 and state the service you require. The operator will need your name and telephone number.

   When you are connected to the emergency service you should give the following information:

1 The exact location of the incident.
2 An indication of the type and seriousness of the incident.
3 Number, sex and age of the casualties.
4 Any extra information for special aid if you suspect a heart attack or childbirth.

First Aid kit

All salons should provide a First Aid box containing a First Aid kit to include, as a minimum: assorted plasters, sterile dressings, bandages (including a triangular bandage), eye pads, scissors, tweezers, safety pins and antiseptic lotion.

   Protective gloves should be provided for use when dealing with wounds which are bleeding or weeping. Unless in an emergency, first aid should not be given without wearing these gloves because of the threat of AIDS.

HEALTH AND INFECTIOUS DISEASE

There are a number of diseases which may be spread in the salon. A knowledge and understanding of these diseases can enable us to be more hygienic and thereby minimize their spread.

Diseases caused by micro-organisms

Micro-organisms are generally so small they cannot be seen without the use of a microscope. There are many different types of micro-organism. Some are harmless (**non-pathogenic**), others may cause disease (**pathogenic**). Pathogens may be bacteria, fungi or viruses.

BACTERIA are single-celled (unicellular) organisms. All bacteria need food, water and warmth and some also need oxygen so that they can grow and reproduce. They do this rapidly when conditions are good, both inside and outside the human body (some can double their numbers in 20-30 minutes). In bad conditions some bacteria can produce resistant spores in which they can survive for long periods until conditions improve. Bacterial infections are treated with antibiotics.

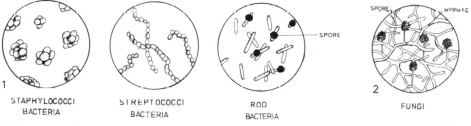

STAPHYLOCOCCI
BACTERIA

STREPTOCOCCI
BACTERIA

ROD
BACTERIA

— SPORE

SPORE   HYPHAE

FUNGI

1 Some examples of bacteria as seen under a light microscope

2 An example of a fungus as seen under a light microscope

FUNGI are non-green plants which form a mass of tangled filaments (hyphae) which together form the body (mycelium) of the fungus. Although the fungus may be visible to the naked eye (e.g. mould on food), the hyphae are microscopic. They need the same sort of growing conditions as bacteria and reproduce by producing large numbers of resistant spores.

VIRUSES are much smaller than bacteria and fungi and cannot be seen even with a light microscope. They are capable of 'life' and reproducing only when they are within a living cell of another plant or animal. Viral diseases do not respond to antibiotics.

	Disease/organism	Description	Notes
B A C T E R I A	Impetigo caused by Streptococci	Blisters on outer epidermis of skin which dry to form a yellow crust.	Bacteria enter through a break in the skin where chapping or scratching has occurred. Highly infectious, especially in children.
	Boils caused by Staphylococci	Infection of hair follicle followed by inflammation and development of pus in hair follicle.	Burn all contaminated dressings etc.
	Barbers' itch (*Sycosis barbae*) caused by Staphylococci.	Infection of hair follicles of beard. Pustules form around each hair.	Transmitted by infected razors, shaving brushes towels, etc.
F U N G I	Ringworm, found in various parts of the body:		Fungus attacks dead tissues of the epidermis and hair shaft.
	Tinea capitis (scalp)	Pink patches on scalp, develop into round grey scaly area with broken hairs.	Highly contagious. Spreads by direct contact. Most common in children.
	Tinea pedis (athlete's foot)	Soggy white patches between toes, later becoming dry and scaly.	Treatment by Griseofulvin.
	Other ringworms include body, nail and beard ringworm.		
V I R U S E S	Colds, flu	Infections of upper respiratory tract — runny or blocked nose, sore throat, cough, etc.	Spread by droplet infection. Very common.
	Cold sores (*Herpes simplex*)	Infection of skin, especially around nose and lips. Periodically forms red, itchy spot which may develop blisters.	Tends to be a life-long infection which erupts every now and again.
	Warts (*Verrucae*)	Small growths on skin.	Cannot be 'cured' but can be 'burnt off' by heat or chemicals.

	Disease/organism	Description	Notes
V **I** **R** **U** **S** **E** **S**	AIDS (Acquired Immune Deficiency Syndrome)	Virus attacks the natural defence system of the body so that the person is unable to fight disease and some cancers. A very serious disease which can lead to death.	Usually transmitted through sex. Can also be transmitted if blood, tissue fluid or semen from an infected person enters a break in the skin of a healthy person.
	Hepatitis B	Virus attacks liver. A very serious disease which can lead to death.	Transmitted by contact with very small amounts of blood or tissue fluid.

Infestation by animal parasites

A parasite is an organism which can only obtain nourishment from another living organism (a host). An attack on the body by small animal parasites is known as an infestation. Infestations can often lead to secondary infections, e.g. impetigo, boils, by micro-organisms entering breaks in the skin caused by scratching or parasite bites. Some parasites are carriers of disease, e.g. lice can carry Typhus fever. All parasitic infections are highly contagious (see page 14).

THE HEAD LOUSE (*PEDICULOSIS CAPITIS*)   Head lice are most likely to be found on the scalp behind the ears, on the sides of the head and on the nape of the neck.

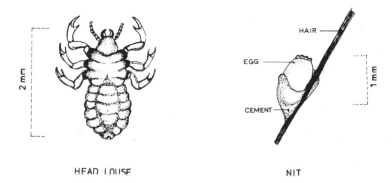

HEAD LOUSE

NIT

The adult lice are grey and about 2 mm long. They can bite the skin and suck blood. The bites cause irritation to the skin and induce scratching. The females lay eggs on the hair close to the scalp, which are cemented to the hair. The eggs are white, oval and about 1 mm long. They are called 'nits'. *Pediculosis* is treated by the use of an insecticide, e.g. Malathion, which kills the lice and the nits. This should be applied by the client at home.

THE ITCH MITE (SCABIES)   Scabies is a contagious skin infestation caused by the itch mite. It does not involve the face and scalp but can occur anywhere else on the body. The itch mite burrows and breeds in the epidermis of the skin causing intense itching.

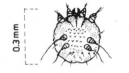

ITCH MITE

ITCH MITE BURROW IN SKIN

HYGIENE

How infection is spread

Micro-organisms are found everywhere and exist in large numbers on the skin, in the nose and mouth, on dirty hairdressing equipment (such as scissors, brushes, combs, etc.), clothing, basins, work surfaces, floors and dust. The close contact between hairdresser and client, the warm and moist atmosphere of the salon and the use of some hairdressing tools on more than one client provide ideal conditions for the spread of infection. Infection may be spread by either direct or indirect contact.

DIRECT CONTACT   A disease transferred by direct contact is **contagious.** It can be spread in two ways:

1   Droplet infection — by inhaling air-borne droplets which have come from the nose or mouth of an infected person.
2   By touching an infected area of the body.

INDIRECT CONTACT   This can take place in three ways:

1   By touching an infected object, e.g. gown, brush, scissors, etc.
2   From infected animals, e.g. lice, fleas, rats and mice.
3   From infected food and water.

Preventing the spread of infection

There are seven important ways through which the spread of infection can be prevented:

1   Clients with skin infections or infestations should not be given hairdressing services but tactfully referred to a doctor. If work has already begun before it is noticed, then the service should be completed as quickly as possible. Contaminated hair should be swept up immediately and burnt. Hairdressing equipment and clothing which has been in contact with the client must be sterilized or disinfected.

2   All work surfaces must be regularly cleaned with hot water and detergent. A daily wipe with surgical spirit is also recommended for most surfaces, but care should be taken not to over-use it on plastic surfaces. Surfaces should be made of materials which are free of cracks and easy to keep clean.

3   Each hairdresser should have at least two sets of tools, one in use and the other being sterilized or disinfected, ready for the next client.

4   Clean gowns (or disposable neck strips) should be given to each client. Towels should be washed and dried after use (not simply dried).

5   Hair should be swept up after every hair cut and burnt at the end of the day.

6   Personal hygiene is important, in particular hands should be washed after visiting the lavatory or blowing the nose.

7   Because of the risk of AIDS and Hepatitis B, care should be taken when using tools which may cut or pierce the skin or where there are open, bleeding or weeping wounds or cuts. These diseases can be passed on by transferring minute amounts of blood from someone with the disease or a carrier of the disease to a healthy person. Combs, brushes, etc. should not be used on broken skin affected with boils, weeping eczema or rashes, unless they can be sterilized immediately afterwards. Disposable razors should be

used once only and then safely thrown away. Scissors or clippers which cut the skin should be immediately washed and sterilized.

Sterilization and disinfection

Sterilization and disinfection techniques may be physical (heat and ultraviolet radiation) or chemical. All tools must be washed with hot water and detergent before disinfection or sterilization is attempted. For AIDS and Hepatitis B, disinfection is not adequate, sterilization is required.

STERLIZATION means the complete destruction of all living organisms.

Autoclaves are highly recommended especially for medium to large salons. Autoclaving is the most efficient method for sterilizing metal objects, combs and plastics. Autoclaves sterilize by the action of heat (steam) and pressure.

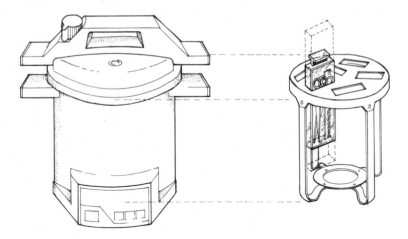

A typical salon autoclave

Boiling in water Where autoclaves are not available, metal objects may be sterilized by boiling in water for 30 minutes. Towels and linens may also be sterilized in this way.

Dry heat Burning completely destroys pathogens. Hair cuttings, soiled dressings, etc. should always be burnt.

Ultraviolet radiation cabinet   Ultraviolet rays (u/v) will kill micro-organisms. The cabinet contains a mercury vapour lamp which produces u/v light. Total sterilization of hairdressing tools is rarely achieved using this technique, therefore the other methods should be used wherever possible. If you *have* to use a u/v radiation cabinet, then remember that the tools must be perfectly clean before u/v irradiation. Any part of the tool which is not in direct contact with the u/v light, e.g. in a shadow or under-side, will not be sterilized. Therefore, allow plenty of space between tools and turn over frequently to expose all surfaces to the rays. Each surface should be irradiated for 20-30 minutes.

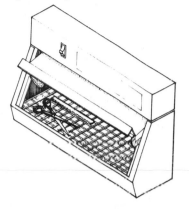

DISINFECTANTS   are chemical substances which will kill most pathogens when used for long enough at sufficiently strong concentrations.

Liquid disinfectants   are germicides and bactericides, e.g. phenolic compounds from coal tar.

Disinfectants are only effective if used correctly. They quickly become stale or overloaded, some are poisonous to humans or corrosive to equipment, and all have to be used at the correct concentration for the correct time, otherwise they will act only as antiseptics. Therefore, when using disinfectants always follow the manufacturer's instructions exactly.

Chemical vapour cabinet   Formaldehyde vapour cabinets can be used to disinfect equipment. However, because of the considerable health hazards associated with the use of formaldehyde its use is strongly discouraged, other techniques are considered preferable.

ANTISEPTICS   are chemicals which are used to reduce the rate at which micro-organisms multiply. An example of an antiseptic is 1% Cetrimide (a quaternary ammonium compound) which is useful as an antiseptic wipe for salon surfaces. If soaps or soapless detergents are mixed with this antiseptic then it will stop working.

Natural immunity

This is the natural ability of the body to combat disease. Special 'white cells' are found in the blood and at the site of an infection. These are able to destroy pathogens by producing antibodies. White cells may also have the ability to destroy pathogens by engulfing them.

FIRE HAZARDS AND PREVENTION

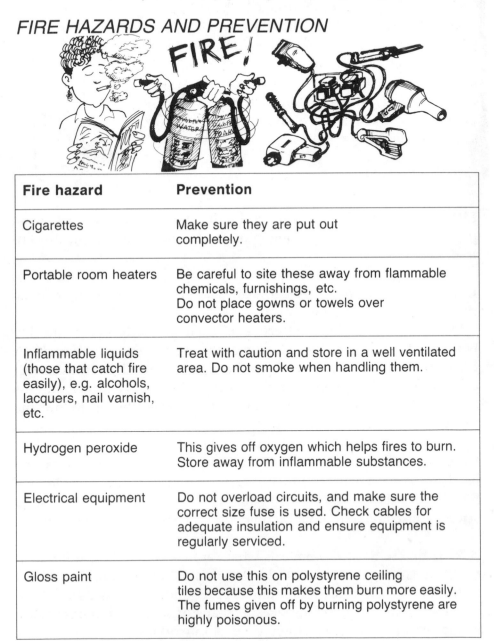

Fire hazard	Prevention
Cigarettes	Make sure they are put out completely.
Portable room heaters	Be careful to site these away from flammable chemicals, furnishings, etc. Do not place gowns or towels over convector heaters.
Inflammable liquids (those that catch fire easily), e.g. alcohols, lacquers, nail varnish, etc.	Treat with caution and store in a well ventilated area. Do not smoke when handling them.
Hydrogen peroxide	This gives off oxygen which helps fires to burn. Store away from inflammable substances.
Electrical equipment	Do not overload circuits, and make sure the correct size fuse is used. Check cables for adequate insulation and ensure equipment is regularly serviced.
Gloss paint	Do not use this on polystyrene ceiling tiles because this makes them burn more easily. The fumes given off by burning polystyrene are highly poisonous.

Dealing with fire in the salon

The Fire Service will be able to advise about fire exits and extinguishers in the salon. All staff should know the fire drill and what to do
in an emergency.

IN THE EVENT OF A FIRE Remember that the safety of people is
more important than anything else. A small fire may be tackled by a
fire extinguisher, but unless it goes out almost immediately, the
building must be evacuated and the Fire Brigade sent for. Remember
to close windows and doors if possible; this helps to stop the spread of
fire.

PUTTING OUT FIRES Deprive the fire of heat, air or material to
burn. There are several types of fire extinguishers available. These are:

1 Water extinguishers which cool the fire. They are acceptable for
   general use but **do not** use on electrical fires (danger of electric
   shock) or burning liquid fires (water may spread the fire even
   further).
2 Sand extinguishers which exclude air from the fire. They can be
   used for burning liquids or electrical fires (turn off electricity first).
3 Carbon dioxide (CO_2) fire extinguishers exclude air from the fire
   and are available in foam or gas form. CO_2 gas is preferred
   because it is less messy and does not conduct electricity.
4 BCF extinguishers (bromochlorodifluoromethane) exclude air from
   the fire and cool the fire. They do not conduct electricity. Smoke
   produced is poisonous, so there must be good ventilation. BCF
   extinguishers do not make any mess or damage furniture.
5 Dry powder extinguishers exclude air from the fire. The powder is
   usually sodium bicarbonate. They have the advantage of being
   easy to clean after use.

ELECTRICITY AND ELECTRICAL SAFETY

An understanding of what electricity is and some of its characteristics
will help you to work with it safely.

Electricity is a form of energy. Two types exist: stationary or static
electricity, and moving or current electricity.

Static electricity

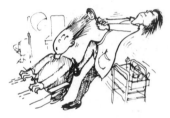

Static electricity is commonly seen on the hair. For example after brushing newly washed hair with a nylon brush, the hairs spring apart and tend to cling to the brush and follow its movements. Static electricity is a build up of electrical charge caused by friction (rubbing two things together) in which the hair becomes positively charged and the brush negatively charged. Since unlike charges attract one another, the hair is attracted to and sticks to the brush.

Current electricity

Substances which allow a flow of electricity through them are known as **conductors,** e.g. silver (the best), copper (very good), most other metals, water. **Insulators** are substances which do not allow the flow of electricity, e.g. rubber, plastic, air, porcelain, dry hair. Electricity will flow through a conductor provided that there is a continuous closed path known as a **circuit.** The flow of electricity through such a circuit is known as **current electricity.**

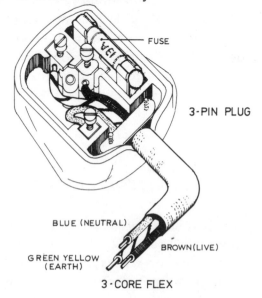

FUSE

3-PIN PLUG

BLUE (NEUTRAL)

BROWN (LIVE)

GREEN YELLOW
(EARTH)

3-CORE FLEX

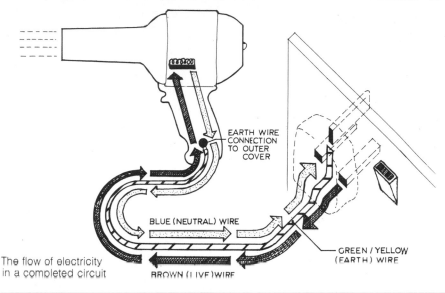

EARTH WIRE
CONNECTION
TO OUTER
COVER

BLUE (NEUTRAL) WIRE

GREEN / YELLOW
(EARTH) WIRE

The flow of electricity
in a completed circuit

BROWN (LIVE) WIRE

An **alternating current** is one in which the direction of electrical flow is reversed many times each second. This is the type of electricity which is supplied to the salon and your home through the mains supply. In a **direct current** the electricity flows in one direction only. This type of electricity is supplied from batteries.

Each electrical appliance must be part of a circuit if it is to work. The electricity flows from the mains into a three-pin plug.

From here electricity passes down the live wire (coloured brown) which is made of copper and insulated by plastic. The neutral wire (blue) can be thought of as returning the electricity to the mains after it has flowed through the appliance, and so completing the circuit. The earth wire (green and yellow) is a safety device which is connected to the outer cover of the electrical appliance so that if any metal parts come into contact with the live wire (and so themselves become 'live', i.e. conduct the electricity), the earth wire conducts this electricity away, preventing the user from getting an electric shock.

All appliances with metal on the outside should be earthed unless they have this sign on them ▣ . This means they are **double insulated** and there is no danger of a fault causing the outside to become 'live'.

Another safety device present in the plug is the **fuse**. This is designed to be the weakest part of the circuit. If the current passing is too large for the circuit, the fuse wire becomes hot and melts thus breaking the circuit and stopping the electric current. The fuse always forms part of the live wire of the circuit.

The electricity is pushed around the circuit by electrical pressure from the mains. This pressure, or strength of pushing, is measured in **volts.** The main supply in this country is 240 volts.

The size of the electric current (how much electricity is flowing round the circuit) is measured in **amps.** The ampage of a circuit will vary according to the power of the appliance within the circuit. Electrical power is measured in **watts.** The higher the wattage the more powerful the appliance, e.g. a 1500 watt hairdryer is more powerful and will dry hair quicker than a 750 watt hairdryer.

A kilowatt (1000 watts) appliance used for one hour uses one kilowatt hour of electricity. This is known as one unit of electricity and is used in the calculation of the cost of electricity.

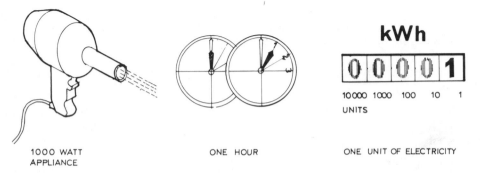

| 1000 WATT APPLIANCE | ONE HOUR | ONE UNIT OF ELECTRICITY |

The outer cover of an electrical appliance should contain information regarding its voltage and wattage. Using this information it is possible to work out the size of the electric current (amps) which would flow in that circuit.

$$\text{Amps} = \frac{\text{watts}}{\text{volts}}$$

CALCULATION OF FUSE SIZE   The ampage of the circuit will determine the size of the fuse which should be contained in the three-pin plug; 3, 5 and 13 amp fuses are in common use.

For example a hairdryer of 700 watts:

$$\text{Amps} = \frac{\text{watts}}{\text{volts}} = \frac{700}{240} = 2.9 \text{ amps}$$

Use a fuse size just bigger than the amps in the circuit; in this case use a 3 amp fuse.

For a hairdryer of 1200 watts:

$$\text{Amps} = \frac{\text{watts}}{\text{volts}} = \frac{1200}{240} = 5 \text{ amps}$$

Therefore use a 5 amp fuse.

For a fan heater of 3000 (3 kw):

$$\text{Amps} = \frac{\text{watts}}{\text{volts}} = \frac{3000}{240} = 12.5 \text{ amps}$$

Therefore use a 13 amp fuse.

It is important to use a fuse size that is just larger than the ampage of the circuit. For example, if a 13 amp fuse is used where a 3 amp fuse would be best, then there is a danger that the circuit could be overloaded without the fuse breaking. This could result in failure of equipment, overheating and the outbreak of a fire.

If several electrical appliances are connected to one power point by means of an adaptor or multi-socket outlet and their combined wattage is greater than that allowed for by the fuse, then the circuit would be overloaded.

For example, if a 1200 w hairdryer and a 60 w light bulb are used in a circuit with a 5 amp fuse:

$$\text{Amps} = \frac{\text{watts}}{\text{volts}} = \frac{1200 + 60}{240} = \frac{1260}{240} = 5.2 \text{ amps}$$

Since the current is greater than the fuse size, the circuit will be overloaded and the fuse will blow.

Other causes of overloading of circuits include faults within the appliance, such as short circuits.

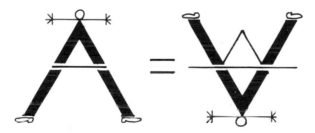

Electric shock

If a person's body completes a mains circuit, electricity will flow through him/her and he/she will experience an electric shock. The size of the shock will depend on the size of the current. It can vary from a feeling of slight tingling to cardiac arrest (where the heart stops beating) and cessation of breathing. A person could become part of an electric circuit in several different ways:

1   By touching bare wires on flexes and cables where insulation is worn or faulty. Any flexes with worn insulation and broken or cracked plugs and switches should be replaced.

2   Through the incorrect wiring or through a fault in the plug or appliance.

3   Through touching a switch or plug with wet hands. The water acts as a good conductor and the electricity may flow through the person rather than the circuit.

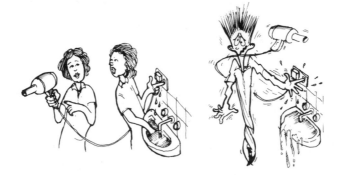

ELECTRIC SHOCK FIRST AID   The person may not be able to break contact with the live apparatus. Do not touch the person unless you are well insulated yourself or you will also get a shock. Switch off the current by removing the plug or by turning the electricity off at the main switch. If breathing has stopped, apply artificial respiration (see First Aid on page 10). This may need to be continued for some time. Seek medical assistance.

MULTIPLE CHOICE QUESTIONS

1 Metal objects such as scissors, combs and plastics can best be sterilized by treatment with:
   (a)   ultraviolet light   (c)   an anionic detergent
   (b)   ammonia   (d)   an autoclave
2 Which of the following fire extinguishers should **not** be used on an electrical fire?
   (a)   carbon dioxide   (c)   water
   (b)   BCF   (d)   dry powder
3 If a client has permanent wave lotion in his or her eye, you should:
   (a)   send him/her to the doctor
   (b)) wipe the eye with a clean tissue
   (c)   wash the eye with running water
   (d)   cover the eye with a sterile eye pad and bandage
4 The first action in the event of someone receiving an electric shock should be to:
   (a)   apply mouth to mouth resuscitation
   (b)   turn off the electricity
   (c)   throw water over them
   (d)   loosen clothing around the neck
5 An antiseptic will:
   (a)   sterilize metal objects
   (b)   kill all known germs
   (c)   reduce the rate at which micro-organisms multiply
   (d)   destroy unpleasant smells
6 An electric current in which the flow is continually reversing is known as:
   (a)   an alternating current   (c)   an eddy current
   (b)   an insulated current   (d)   a direct current
7 The colour of the insulation around the live wire in a modern flex is:
   (a)   green and yellow   (c)   red
   (b)   brown   (d)   black
8 Suitable fuse sizes can be calculated from:
   (a) $\dfrac{\text{watts}}{\text{volts}}$

   (b)   volts x watts
   (c) $\dfrac{\text{amps}}{\text{volts}}$

   (d)   amps x watts

9 If a hand-held hairdryer is not double insulated, it must be fitted with an earth wire to:
   (a) control the temperature
   (b) bring the current from the mains
   (c) help prevent electric shock in the event of a fault
   (d) complete the circuit

10 An example of a good insulator is:
   (a) plastic
   (b) copper
   (c) silver
   (d) water

11 *Pediculosis* is treated by the use of:
   (a) an antiseptic cream
   (b) Griseofulvin
   (c) antibiotics
   (d) Malathion

12 For a burn of the hand:
   (a) smear butter over affected area
   (b) hold under running cold water
   (c) cover with sticking plaster
   (d) apply an antiseptic

13 A short circuit may be caused by:
   (a) a flex that is too short
   (b) a blown mains fuse
   (c) faulty insulation
   (d) overloading the circuit

14 An example of a skin disorder caused by a fungus is:
   (a) impetigo
   (b) psoriasis
   (c) a wart
   (d) ringworm

15 Which one of the following may enforce the Health and Safety at Work Act:
   (a) the police
   (b) Health and Safety Inspectors
   (c) Customs and Excise Officers
   (d) Department of Health and Social Security employees.

3
PERSONAL PRESENTATION

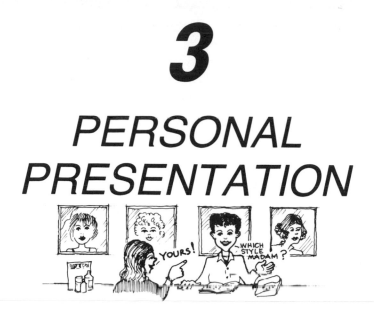

CREATING A GOOD IMPRESSION

There are many hairdressing salons. How do clients choose which one to go to? Clients notice their friends' and neighbours' hairstyles and often ask where they have their hair done, whilst others are attracted by the outside shop fronts or a good reception display. When clients enter the salon they must be made to feel happy and relaxed. Most people look quite unattractive with wet hair, combed flat to their heads, and so often feel ill at ease in a hairdressing salon. However, if you the hairdresser can give clients confidence in whichever service is being carried out they will return to *your* salon.

If clients like the way that the hairdresser is dressed and like the hairdresser's own hairstyle, then they will have even more confidence in their own finished hairstyle. This is why large photographs of styles done by hairstylists working in the salon encourage clients to try out new looks.

Hairdressers must be alert and must try to understand the client's needs and wishes. It is the job of the hairdresser to help clients to select a style that is suitable for them — for their hair, scalp and skin condition (see Chapter 5), as well as personality and life-style. This analysis should be done every time the client visits the salon as a client's needs may change from time-to-time. For example, a woman may need a hair style for a special occasion such as a dinner/dance, or a man may have changed his job and need a more fashionable hair style.

If the hairdresser looks presentable, i.e. neat, well-groomed and clean, then the client will have more confidence and is likely to return to your salon time and time again.

PERSONAL WELL-BEING

Hairdressing is a very tiring profession and standing on your feet all day, bending your back and keeping a smile on your face, is very difficult! A good diet, regular exercise and sufficient sleep helps everyone to lead a good life, but if you are a hairdresser it is vital.

A BALANCED DIET The body needs nutrients to provide the raw materials for growth and repair, to give it energy and to protect it against disease. These raw materials are obtained from the food we eat. The body needs carbohydrates (contained in sweet and starchy foods) and fats (contained in oily or fatty foods) to provide energy. Proteins contained in meat, fish, eggs, beans and nuts) enable us to grow or repair ourselves. Vitamins and minerals are needed in very small amounts but are essential for good health. In order to obtain all of these you should eat a variety of foods, including fresh fruit and vegetables. It is also very important to drink plenty of liquids, preferably water, each day.

GOOD POSTURE is important too, not only because it looks better, as clothes will hang properly, but because it is more healthy since the bones, muscles, tendons and ligaments will be held in their correct position. This avoids undue stretching and strain.

To stand correctly

In order to stand correctly the weight of the body should be carried equally on both legs. Hips and shoulders should be level and the head held up. Common faults are round shoulders, hollow back and weight held mostly on one foot so that the shoulders and hips are tilted.

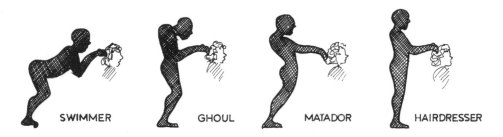

SWIMMER   GHOUL   MATADOR   HAIRDRESSER

To sit correctly

In order to sit correctly the bones should form a right-angle at the hip and knee, with the hips and most of the thighs supported by the chair. Common faults are slouching, (only the base of the spine is in contact with the chair so that the back and thighs are not supported) and crossing the legs.

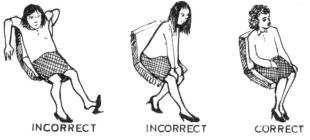

INCORRECT   INCORRECT   CORRECT

REGULAR EXERCISE All muscles need to be worked if they are to remain healthy. If unused, muscles will begin to weaken and waste away. Regular exercise, e.g. running, swimming and aerobics, will keep the muscles working correctly and help to maintain a good body shape. Exercise will also improve respiration, digestion and blood circulation, as well as relaxing nervous tension.

SUFFICIENT SLEEP The body needs sleep in order that the nervous system can function efficiently but, the amount of sleep needed varies from person to person. Lack of sleep causes irritability, lack of concentration and clumsy body movements. It is not a good idea to tell the manager that you have spilled the client's coffee over her because you were out at the disco all night!

SUFFICIENT RELAXATION Rest is necessary when the body needs to stop using certain parts which have been working hard, in order to allow them to recover. The work can either be physical or mental, and rest can be taken in the form of relaxation or sleep or change of activity.

THE ABILITY TO COPE WITH STRESS Stress can be caused by a variety of different factors, including boredom, emotional strain, lack of sleep, repetitive tasks such as daily routines, or overcrowding and hot humid conditions e.g. in a busy salon. Think how often people in a salon become irritated and cross for no particular reason. Stress in a salon is often not caused by difficult clients but by these other factors.

Personal cleanliness

Personal cleanliness is essential for good health and also to avoid giving offence because of bad breath or body odour. Think how close you stand to clients whilst doing their hair! The skin can be kept clean by washing with soap and water to remove dirt, unwanted skin (epidermal) scales, sebum (see page 68) and stale sweat. These all provide breeding grounds for germs which can cause disease or body odour. Deodorants (which mask smells) and antiperspirants (which reduce sweating) can also help to prevent body odour. Washing also helps to prevent the pores of the skin from becoming blocked, which can result in blackheads and spots.

Make-up should be removed from the skin by using cold-cream or cleanser, because these are fatty emulsions (see page 52) which stick to make-up. These mixtures can be wiped off with a tissue or cotton wool. Skin toners or astringents (e.g. cold water, witch-hazel, after-shave lotions) may be applied to close the pores and tighten the skin. Moisturisers can be used on the face, hands or body for dry skin or to overcome the drying effects of chemicals in soap or detergents.

Personal appearance

Remember, a client's first impression of you is lasting.

SKIN TYPES   There are several different types of skin. These range from normal, greasy or oily, or dry, to combination (greasy forehead, nose and chin, but dry cheeks), and sensitive. The skin problem of acne (*acne vulgaris*) may be sometimes caused by a hormone imbalance. Make sure that you use the correct cleanser, moisturiser and toner for your skin type. Manufacturers now produce ranges for men as well as women.

EYEBROWS   Use tweezers to shape eyebrows when and if necessary.

FEATURES   There are several different face shapes (see p. 260). These vary from oval, round, square, or oblong, to heart, diamond or triangular shapes.

SKIN COLOUR   Skin also varies from person to person. It may be red (florid), grey (sallow) or pink (healthy skin) and there may be broken capillaries on the cheeks.

MAKE-UP   cosmetics worn during the day for work are generally softer than those worn in the evening because of different lighting. Paler make-up looks good in daylight but stronger colours are needed under artificial light in the evening.

FOUNDATION   Foundations may be liquid, cream, gel or stick. They are applied to the face and neck to give a uniform, matt appearance to the skin and to cover any blemishes. It is a good idea to try the colour first on the inside of your wrist to see if it matches your skin tone.

FACE POWDER   Face powder may be loose and applied with a brush, or compact and applied with a sponge. It is used on top of foundation to give a matt appearance.

BLUSHER   This is used on or around the cheekbones to highlight or lowlight the features. It must be well blended in with a brush or make-up sponge.

CONTOUR PRODUCTS An oval face shape is considered to be perfect. Other face shapes may be improved by clever make-up. Lighter shades can be used on certain areas to enhance features, e.g. high cheekbones, or darker shades can hide other areas, e.g. a square jawline.

CONCEALER STICKS These are heavier versions of foundation, and are used to conceal blemishes or unwanted shading (e.g. bags under the eyes).

EYESHADOW Eyeshadows are used to accentuate the eyes. They can come in powder, cream, gels, liquid or lotion form. Generally, protruding eyes need darker colours and deep-set eyes need lighter colours. *Fashion,* however, often dictates the colour of the day.

EYELINER AND EYE PENCIL These may be liquid or crayon and are used inside or outside the eyelashes to emphasise the eye shape.

MASCARA Mascara is used to darken and lengthen eyelashes in order to make them appear more luxurious. It may be block and brush, spiral or comb brush, waterproof, lash-lengthening or non-allergic. Several applications may be needed to achieve thickness and body, and it may be applied to both upper and lower lashes.

LIPSTICK Most women wear lipstick and sometimes lip gloss for extra shine. Lip liner is used to outline the shape of the mouth. Dark colours will make the lips appear smaller and are useful for large lips, whereas light colours have the effect of making the lips look larger and are, therefore, best on small lips.

Most people can wear different shades to match their outfits, but it is a good idea to remember that orange shades draw attention to sallow skins and pale colours draw attention to poor teeth and bad skin.

BEARDS Beards should be kept neat and regularly trimmed. Before shaving, the skin is prepared by applying shaving foam, either from an aerosol or by the bowl and brush method, to raise the bristles. The beard growth may then be removed by using an open razor. Many men use an electric shaver which needs no shaving foam. To obtain a clean shave it must be cut both with and against the growth of the beard.

If the skin is nicked or cut, then a liquid or powder stypic (a substance which stops the bleeding) may be applied to the wound.

Aftershave is normally applied after shaving, once the shaving foam and beard stubble is removed from the skin, in order to close the pores and give a refreshing feeling.

HAIR CARE A hairdresser's hair always reflects the standard of the salon. It must be shampooed and conditioned, brushed and combed, regularly. Each salon likes to project a certain image. Does your hairstyle reflect the image of your salon?

TEETH Teeth should be cleaned after meals to remove food particles which provide a breeding ground for bacteria. These can produce dental caries (tooth decay), infection of the gums and bad breath. Dental floss should be used in addition to a toothbrush and is especially made to clean between the teeth after brushing, to remove any remaining food.

Sometimes stomach disorders or simply eating strongly flavoured foods, such as curries or garlic, can result in breath smelling for some time. Breath fresheners are often available in tablet or spray forms and need to be used if this is the case.

Regular visits to the dentist will ensure that teeth are kept clean and stain-free, and any dental repairs such as fillings can be done at the same time.

HANDS As a hairdresser your hands are the tools of your trade — so look after them!

Clients see your hands working in the mirror all the time, so both hands and nails must be perfectly clean. Hairdressers often suffer from dry hands because of harsh chemicals and constant immersion in water or working with wet hair. Keep hand cream and barrier cream near you, and use it constantly. Cuts and abrasions and rough skin can lead to contact dermatitis (eczema) and infections (see Chapter 2), so they must be dealt with immediately.

NAILS Some nail disorders are caused by allergies to nail varnish (enamel), whilst others are caused by infections. It is important to know the difference and which need medical attention in order to prevent the spread of infection: e.g. Whitlows (infection of the cuticle), and ingrown nails (nails growing into the skin).

Nails should be cut, filed and shaped regularly so that they do not catch in the client's hair or scratch the client's scalp. Split, flaking, ridged, bitten, stained and hang nails may all be attended to by regular manicures.

If nail varnish is worn in the salon, it must never be chipped. It should be removed with nail varnish remover (acetone, ethyl acetate).

FEET   As hairdressers stand all day long, uncomfortable feet can be unbearable! Hard skin, e.g. callouses and corns, are caused by shoes constantly rubbing, so make sure your shoes fit properly for work. It is dangerous to wear sandals or open-toed shoes in the salon because sharp razors and scissors may be dropped, and cut hairs can easily embed themselves under skin and toenails.

Feet sweat in the salon so wash them regularly and dry them properly, especially between the toes. Athlete's Foot is a painful condition where the skin flakes and becomes sore, but can be rectified by using appropriate foot creams and powders (see page 12).

Some foot disorders do need proper medical care: e.g. veruccas, ingrowing toenails and bunions.

Toenails must be cut (preferably straight across), and filed regularly. A regular pedicure, complete with well applied nail varnish helps feet to look good and well cared for.

CLOTHES   A hairdresser's style of dress reflects attitudes to fashion and the design of the salon. Accessories such as jewellery, including earrings, brooches, hair ornaments and badges, must blend with the overall look. Too much jewellery can look out of place and catch in the client's hair, and in tools and equipment.

An appreciation of design, including colour and patterns, is given in Chapter 15.

Generally, clothes worn in the salon should be comfortably loose fitting, clean, neatly pressed and regularly mended. Cotton fabrics are often cooler to wear, but synthetics are generally more hard-wearing. All clothes are expensive to buy, so it is always sensible to wear dye aprons when using hair-colours and bleaches.

INTER-PERSONAL SKILLS

Your appearance and ability to communicate (by verbal or non-verbal means) as well as your hairdressing skills add up to make you a 'professional'. Good communications can promote a happy atmosphere amongst staff and between staff and clients.

Remember successful salons make money, this is necessary for both the staff and for the salon's growth, for example to buy new equipment and redecorate, or to employ more staff.

Non-verbal communication

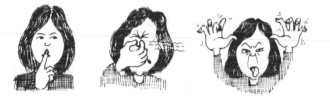

Smiling at others encourages good humour and a pleasant manner. It is very difficult not to smile back at someone who smiles at you!

Non-verbal communication also means using eye contact, i.e. looking into someone's eyes whilst speaking to them to gain their confidence.

Gestures, particularly hand movements, are often used to express feelings, but hairdressers must not overdo it. Remember you may have a pair of scissors in your hands at the time!

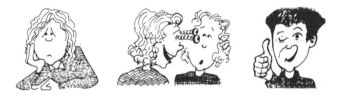

Posture or stance are just as important as clothes. A slovenly appearance can be very off-putting.

Verbal communication

Speaking clearly and politely is very important. Have you ever listened to yourself speak on a tape-recorder? Your tone of voice, high or low pitch of speaking, how fast you talk and how loudly you speak often comes as a complete surprise. If you see yourself on a video recording then your body language (i.e. eye contact, gestures and posture) is combined with your speech and you can see yourself as others see you.

Salons often present fashion shows, sometimes for charity, and need to record them on video in order to improve the presentation next time. You may, therefore, find yourself unwittingly on video, and although it may be a shock, try to criticize yourself and see how you could improve.

Hairdressers have to converse with each other and with their clients. It is essential to develop a sense of tact. Bad atmospheres can often be created by a slip of the tongue, e.g. 'my goodness you do have bad dandruff!' The expression on the other person's face could tell you that that particular remark was not welcome!

Confidentiality is also vital, for instance if a client happened to suffer from headlice, the worst thing you could do would be to tell any other clients. Not only would clients worry that they might catch them, but gossip soon spreads.

The giving and receiving of instructions needs to be thought about too. Instructions may be passed from client to hairdresser, between staff (who teach and instruct each other) or from manufacturers' technicians who explain new products and their uses. Take time to think about what you are going to say or listen to and make sure you have understood what you have been told.

Many clients never return to salons perhaps because they may have had a lovely new hairstyle, but it was not the one they asked for! Alternatively, many perms have become frizzy or straight, or hair colours turned green simply because hairdressers have not listened to instructions.

Information is often received over the telephone as well as through face-to-face contact. Using the telephone is a practiced skill, as is using a telephone answering machine. Many people are worried about using these machines simply because they are unprepared. Listen carefully to the message, normally it only asks you to leave your name and telephone number, and to state the enquiry that you are making.

When using the telephone, not only must you have a pleasant manner, but you must give clear, logical, information. So think before you speak. Misunderstandings, e.g. the client booked in for the wrong time or the wrong service, happen when people are in too much of a hurry. Any information must be written down clearly (print if your handwriting is difficult to read), and checked by repeating it to the client.

Most written information is made at the reception area, but sometimes accidents happen in the salon. Again, listen to the person asking for help and decide how bad the accident is. Some people create a dreadful fuss for no real reason, whilst others can have serious problems (e.g. a child drinking an unmarked bottle of hydrogen peroxide, thinking it was a soft drink) and speedy action may be necessary. All accidents, must be written down clearly in the accident register (see page 5 and 6) and an insurance claim form may need to be completed.

Selling skills

Manufacturers employ technical staff to increase the hairdresser's product knowledge. Without this, hairdressers would be less able to sell services or products to their clients.

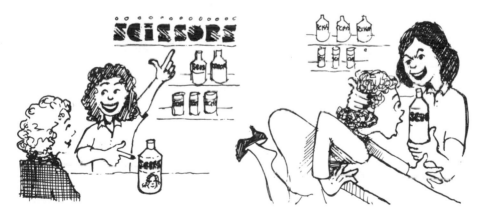

Only when hairdressers are confident with the products that they are selling can they become enthusiastic and effective sales people.

Misinformed opinion can often form a barrier to selling products (even though the hairdresser may receive money commissions on the sales). For example, you may feel that a client may benefit from a permanent wave on their hair, but a friend has said that *all* perms make hair go frizzy. It is then up to the hairdresser to use product knowledge, and perhaps to allow the client to feel someone's hair that has had a good perm, to convince the client that this is not always the case.

Hard selling is when the hairdresser may say for instance, 'would you like a perm on your hair, now?' Soft selling is when the client is allowed time to think about it, for example, 'my hair has been easy to manage with this perm, I'm sure that yours would be, too'.

ADVERTISING   Advertising is a necessary part of selling and can take the form of displays, show cards, fashion shows or staff personal presentation.

Design plays a major role in advertising, and the use of colour, shape and pattern is explained in Chapter 15.

Time, effort and money spent on good advertising is never wasted. Many salons have special promotions, for example reduced prices for hair-colours or highlights, during slack periods of the year such as after Christmas.

Team work

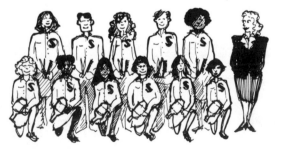

Most salons employ more than one person, and for the salon to run smoothly it is important that people help each other and work as a *team*. The people in a salon will have different skills. Some will be good at cutting, others at perming or colouring, whilst some will be good at all practical skills but may be weak at verbal communication.

Salons must be clean and well organised to work properly and, therefore, junior or back-up staff are just as important as senior members of staff. Good atmospheres are created by positive attitudes and by staff enjoying working together.

Bad atmospheres can be caused by bad behaviour such as rudeness, bad temper, indifference, carelessness and arrogance. New staff are often worried about the unknown, for instance where products are kept in the salon or how to use certain pieces of equipment. Remember your first day? It was probably quite traumatic simply because you did not know anyone and everything was unfamiliar. **Always** be kind and patient with new employees.

Always respond constructively to instructions, criticisms and appraisals — you will be surprised how often it is for your own good! Sometimes it is difficult to tell when someone is being assertive, for example, 'Take Mrs Brown to the basin, now!' or when they are being aggressive, for example, 'Why didn't you take Mrs Brown to the basin when I asked you to?' Stop and think about why the other person behaved in that way. Perhaps it was because they were in a hurry and other clients were being kept waiting. Often the criticism is not being directed at you, but at the situation at the time. Your reaction to every situation is very important, make sure it is always positive.

Likewise, if someone is from a different ethnic origin to you they may not understand the language that you are using. Be patient, and explain yourself again, perhaps using more carefully chosen words the next time. A happy team of salon staff will be appreciated by the clients and they will return again and again!

Professional attitude

Hairdressers should be professional people, which means being impartial and respecting confidentiality, and as such you must always react with tact, courtesy, patience, good humour and a pleasant manner. This is a tall order, especially since it is such a tiring profession!

Individual staff will inspire confidence in others if they are themselves confident, well organized and always punctual. Nothing disrupts a salon more than a member of staff who is consistently late, as clients may be kept waiting.

Remember that whatever personal feelings you have about some-one, (and some clients can be very awkward at times) you must **never** show it. If a situation does become unbearable, it may be wise to excuse yourself for a moment, go away and calm down, and then return with a smile on your face! Clients that have been upset never return to the salon, but the staff have to remain there, so think before you act or speak.

Good relationships in the salon will result in satisfied clients and the potential for increased custom.

MULTIPLE CHOICE QUESTIONS

1 The two major nutrients from which the body gains energy are:
   (a) carbohydrates and fats
   (b) fats and vitamins
   (c) carbohydrates and proteins
   (d) vitamins and minerals

2 Good standing posture is important for a hairdresser because it:
   (a) reduces bone ache
   (b) reduces perspiration
   (c) reduces wear and tear on clothes
   (d) reduces strain on muscles, ligaments and tendons

3 The main purpose of a deodorant is to:
   (a) retard the growth of bacteria
   (b) control perspiration
   (c) destroy offensive odours
   (d) give a pleasant aroma

4 Skin toners or astringents are used:
   (a) to close the pores and tighten the skin
   (b) to remove make-up
   (c) as a skin perfume
   (d) as a foundation cream

5 Sandals should not be worn in the salon because:
   (a) foot odours may be offensive to clients
   (b) they induce bad posture
   (c) the feet may be damaged by falling scissors or cut hairs
   (d) the feet may become cold

6 Which one of the following foods is the best source of protein?
   (a) oranges   (c) cabbage
   (b) fish   (d) wholemeal bread

7 Liquid/powder, stypics are used to:
   (a) give a matt appearance to the face
   (b) soften the beard before shaving
   (c) conceal spots and blemishes
   (d) stop bleeding

8 Cold cream or cleansers are able to remove make-up because:
   (a) cosmetics are fatty emulsions which will stick to them
   (b) they penetrate deep into the pores
   (c) they contain soapless detergents
   (d) they contain soaps

4

SALON PROCEDURES

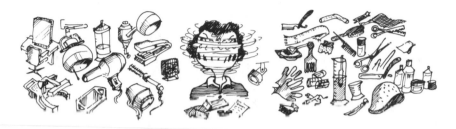

It is important that anyone who works in the salon can identify each piece of equipment and all of the materials used (i.e. products). Mistakes can easily happen!

HAIRDRESSING EQUIPMENT

Equipment	Description/function
Dressing tables	Dressing tables with mirrors are important so that the client may look at her/his reflection.
Dressing chairs	These must be hardwearing, comfortable for the client, the correct height for the hairdresser, and able to withstand chemical spillage.
Mirrors Back mirrors	These are for holding up behind the client to show her the back of her hair.
Plane mirrors	Dressing and backview mirrors have flat surfaces and produce an image which is the same size as the object being viewed.

Concave mirrors

These are curved mirrors which produce an image which may be bigger or smaller than the viewed object. For example, shaving and make-up mirrors are inwardly curving and produce a bigger or magnified image.

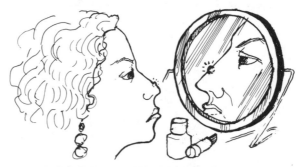

CONCAVE – MAKE-UP MIRROR

Convex mirrors

These are outwardly curving and produce a smaller image over a wider area, e.g. mirrors used in shops to view the whole shopping area.

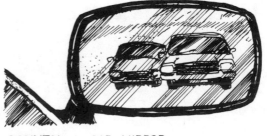

CONVEX – CAR MIRROR

Equipment trolleys

These contain various shapes of trays for holding and storing different equipment. They must always be kept clean, neat and tidy.

Hair dryers

These can be hand held (blow dryers) or free standing (hood dryers). Professional hand dryers are much faster and often heavier to hold than ones for home use. They have automatic temperature controls, so if they become too hot this means that they are faulty and must be checked.

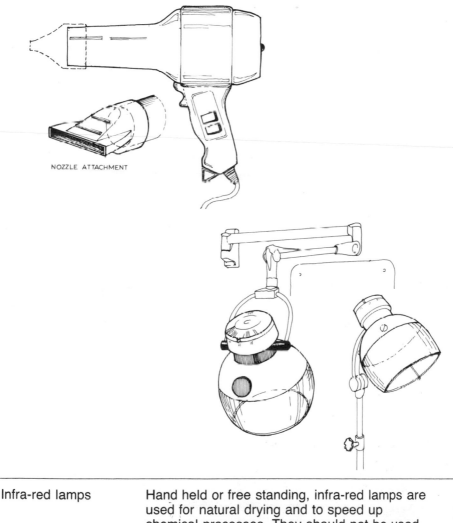

NOZZLE ATTACHMENT

Infra-red lamps

Hand held or free standing, infra-red lamps are used for natural drying and to speed up chemical processes. They should not be used too close to the scalp as they can cause severe scalp burns. The glass round infra-red bulb is fragile and expensive to replace — so take care.

| Accelerators | These are similar to a hood dryer with an infra-red lamp inside. |

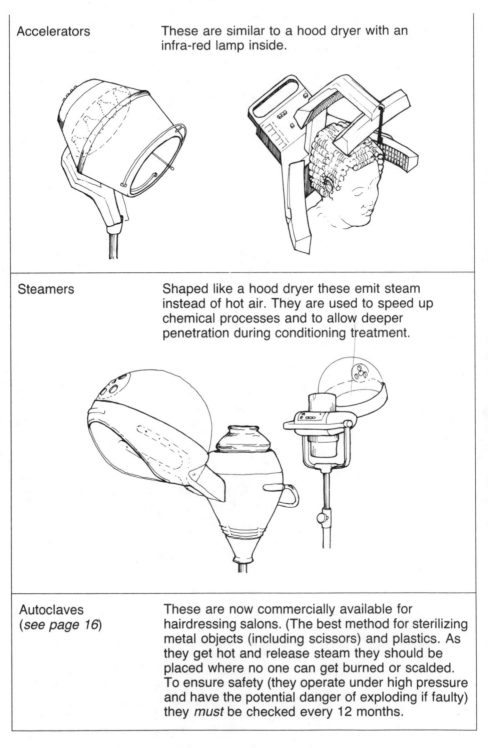

| Steamers | Shaped like a hood dryer these emit steam instead of hot air. They are used to speed up chemical processes and to allow deeper penetration during conditioning treatment. |

| Autoclaves (*see page 16*) | These are now commercially available for hairdressing salons. (The best method for sterilizing metal objects (including scissors) and plastics. As they get hot and release steam they should be placed where no one can get burned or scalded. To ensure safety (they operate under high pressure and have the potential danger of exploding if faulty) they *must* be checked every 12 months. |

Sterilizing cabinet (*see page 17*)	Ultra violet cabinets glow purple when in use. It is difficult to achieve sterilization using them. Chemical sterilizing cabinets should not be used since they give off a strong and dangerous odour when working.

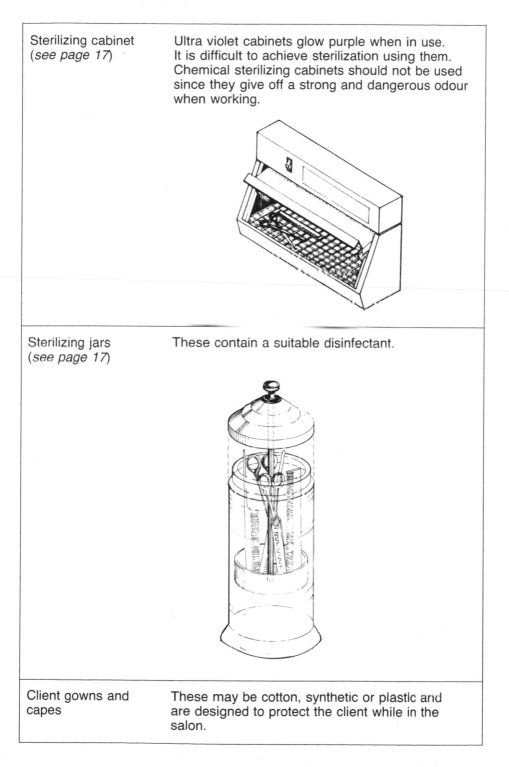

Sterilizing jars (*see page 17*)	These contain a suitable disinfectant.

Client gowns and capes	These may be cotton, synthetic or plastic and are designed to protect the client while in the salon.

Towels	Must be of a size suitable to cover the client's wet hair or to sit comfortably around the shoulders.
Permanent wave bowls (*see Chapter 10*)	These should contain a sufficient amount of perm lotion for one application.
Permanent wave brushes	Lotions are mostly applied direct from small bottles with a nozzle, but a small brush may be used.
Permanent wave sponges (*see Chapter 10*)	These may also be used to apply permanent wave lotion — but **must** be kept separate from neutralizer sponges which usually have a small handle.
Permanent wave curlers or rods (*see Chapter 10*)	These are usually solid and come in various colours and sizes. They are attached to the hair with special rubbers.
End papers (*see Chapter 10*)	These are folded around the ends of the hair to give a smooth finish during winding.
Plastic caps (*see Chapter 10*)	These are used during chemical processes to retain the heat from the head.
Tinting bowls (non-metallic) (*see Chapter 12*)	These should contain a sufficient amount of tint or bleach for one application.
Tinting brushes	Flat brushes used to apply tint or bleach to small sub-sections of hair.
Bleaching caps and hooks (*see Chapter 12*)	These are used to cover the scalp area, and then small meshes of hair are pulled through with the hook and coloured or bleached.
Protective gloves	Worn by the hairdresser these are usually made of rubber and are close fitting to protect the hands during chemical processes.
Hair nets (*see Chapter 7*)	These are used for keeping rollers, pins and clips in place during setting.

Ear Shields (*see Chapter 7*)	These are used to cover the client's ears during drying under a hood dryer. Often paper ear shields are used because they can be thrown away after use.
Cotton wool (*see Chapter 10*)	This is usually in strips to absorb excess chemicals during chemical processes.
Rollers (*see Chapter 7*)	These come in various sizes and colours and are used to produce different effects during setting.
Pins (*see Chapter 7*)	These are used to hold rollers in place.
Clips (*see Chapter 7*)	These are often used for pin curl setting.
Grips (*see Chapter 7*)	These are used to grip hair in dressing techniques — often for long hair.
Butterfly clips (*see Chapter 7*)	These are used to hold large sub-sections of hair during perming or colouring.
Scissors (*see Chapter 8*)	Hairdressing scissors are expensive and finely engineered, and should be looked after.
Thinning scissors (or Aesculaps) (*see Chapter 8*)	These are used to thin hair out.
Razors (*see Chapter 8*)	These may be open (cut-throat) or safety with a guard.
Clippers (*see Chapter 8*)	These are used for short hair cuts and close finishes
Brushes Hair (*see Chapter 7*)	Hair brushes may be made of synthetic (plastic) or natural bristle and may be flat, curved or circular, and of various sizes. The bristles may be open- or close-tufted because they have different uses, e.g. blow-drying, disentangling, disrupting the pli (set) or for dressing out (styling). Pure bristle brushes are kinder to the hair and cause less damage.
Clothes	Clothes brushes (close-tufted) are needed to remove excess hair from the client's clothes.

Neck (*see Chapter 8*)	These are very soft and are used to remove cut hairs from the neck and shoulders during haircutting.
Combs (*see Chapter 7*)	Combs are generally made of vulcanite or plastic and must not have sharp teeth that could graze the client's scalp.
Tail	These are used for setting and sectioning.
Pintail	These are used for permanent wave winding.
Setting (salon comb)	These are used for dressing out, cutting, sectioning, finger waving.
Cutting	A flexible comb used for very short hair work.
Rake	These are used for disentangling wet hair.
Metal comb	These are used for blow waving in gentlemen's hairdressing.
Tongs, hot brushes, crimping irons, heated rollers (*see Chapter 7*)	These are all used on dry hair to create a variety of different effects.

Metal equipment in the salon is often made of anodized steel as this does not react with chemical lotions. Non-professional metal equipment bought from retail shops is often inferior and can turn the client's hair strange colours, e.g. mauve.

HAIRDRESSING MATERIALS

Shampoos (*see Chapter 6*)	These may be thick or thin liquids, paste or powder and often have added perfumes and ingredients, e.g. almond, beer.
Conditioners (*see Chapter 9*)	These may be surface acting, e.g. anti-oxy (anti-oxidation) or deep penetrating, e.g. restructurants.
Oxidizers (*see Chapter 10*)	Neutralizers or normalizers are used after a permanent wave is processed to reform the hair in its new shape.
Setting lotions (*see Chapter 7*)	These may be plain or with added colours and may have extra ingredients for greasy or dry hair. They are often available in individual application sizes.

Mousse and aerosols (*see Chapter 7*)	These may be plain or with added colour and are used for setting, blow drying or natural drying.
Gels (*see Chapter 7*)	These are used for setting, blow drying, or sculpting hair in strong shapes, e.g. wet looks. Gels to add colour or glitter are also used.
Hair spray or lacquers (*see Chapter 7*)	These are used to give hair extra hold whilst finishing the style.
Dressing creams (*see Chapter 7*)	These may be in a cream or aerosol form and used to give extra shine to dry hair.
Hair colourants (*see Chapter 11*)	These are available in bottles (liquid) or tubes (creams). Semi-permanent colours are not mixed with hydrogen peroxide; permanent colours are mixed with hydrogen peroxide.
Skin stain removers (*see Chapter 11*)	These are liquids or creams used to remove hair colouring stains from the client's skin.
Hydrogen peroxide (*see Chapter 12*)	This may be in cream or liquid form, or occasionally powder, and comes in different strengths, e.g. 6% (20 vol.), 9% (30 vol.) and 12% (40 vol.).
Bleach (*see Chapter 12*)	This may be liquid, cream, oil, powder or emulsion and is always mixed with hydrogen peroxide. Some bleaches have sachets of boosters added to them for extra strength.
Permanent wave lotions (*see Chapter 10*)	These are available in large and small bottles and sometimes sachets of chemicals are added to them during use. Different strengths of perm lotion are used on various types of hair, e.g. normal, tinted or bleached.
Hair straighteners (*see Chapter 10*)	These are creams, gels or liquids which are used to chemically straighten curly hair.
Cleaning agents	For example methylated spirits, domestic bleach, proprietary cleaning agents, antiseptic solutions, detergents. **Note:** Domestic bleach is not the same as the bleach used on hair (hydrogen peroxide). It must never be used on the hair or skin since it can cause severe damage.

Storing equipment and materials

All materials and equipment must be stored properly and safely to prevent breakage and wastage. Equipment must always be checked before use, e.g. for frayed flexes on hand dryers, and the correct amount of equipment, both in use and in the stock room, must be controlled.

All the materials listed in the table must be carefully stored, preferably in a cool, dark room. They should all be dated, and old stock must be used first to prevent wastage. The amount of materials used must be priced for each client, e.g. extra perm lotion for long hair will be added to the client's bill, as would retail products sold to the client.

Materials must be carefully measured out to ensure a correct result and for economy. Stock levels (making sure the salon does not run out of anything) are usually controlled by a senior member of staff or sometimes by manufacturer's representatives (Sales Reps).

Each working area in the salon must be continuously re-stocked with the appropriate equipment and materials, e.g. one can of mousse and hair spray to each working area.

NECESSARY SCIENCE

The nature of matter

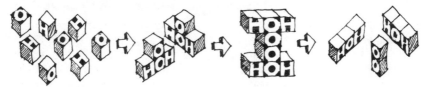

All matter is composed of very small units called **molecules.** Molecules are composed of a number of **atoms.** The chemical formula of a substance tells us what atoms are contained within its molecules:

For example in water (H_2O) one molecule of water consists of two hydrogen atoms (H_2) and one oxygen atom (O).

With oxygen gas (O_2) one molecule of oxygen gas consists of two oxygen atoms (O_2).

With carbon dioxide gas (CO_2) one molecule of carbon dioxide gas consists of one carbon atom (C) and two oxygen atoms (O_2).

There are approximately 105 different types of atoms — each different type is called an **element.**

Elements are the simplest substances which exist. They cannot be split up by any known chemical change into anything more simple.

Atoms of different elements can combine together in chemical reactions to form **compounds,** e.g. water (H_2O), carbon dioxide (CO_2), hydrogen peroxide (H_2O_2) and Keratin, the hair protein, which is a complex compound, containing the elements carbon (C), oxygen (O), hydrogen (H), nitrogen (N) and sulphur (S). The elements within the compound are tightly stuck together by **chemical bonds** and they cannot be separated without breaking these bonds through a chemical reaction. This results in new substances being formed. A **chemical change,** therefore, involves the breaking and reforming of chemical bonds, e.g. hydrogen peroxide easily enters into a chemical reaction, and in so doing forms the new substances water and oxygen.

Two molecules of hydrogen peroxide → two molecules water + one of oxygen

$$2H_2O_2 \quad \rightarrow \quad 2H_2O \quad + \quad O_2$$

Chemical changes are not easily reversed so hairdressing processes which involve chemical changes are usually permanent, e.g. tinting, bleaching, perming.

Molecules of different substances may be mixed together to form a **mixture.** This however does not involve a chemical reaction and the different substances are, therefore, fairly easy to separate. This is known as a **physical change,** e.g. salt and water → salt water. The salt and water may be easily separated, for example by boiling the water away (the salt will be left behind).

Physical changes are easily reversed as no chemical reactions occur and no new chemical compounds are formed. Various physical changes occur during hairdressing processes, e.g. setting, conditioning, wetting, drying (evaporation) and the use of temporary colours.

Solutions

When a substance dissolves in a liquid a **solution** is made (this is a physical change). The substance which dissolves is called the **solute** and the liquid which it dissolves in is called the **solvent.** Many solutions are used in hairdressing, e.g. shampoo — water (solvent) plus soapless detergent (solute); setting lotion — alcohol (solvent) plus plastic resin (solute); perm lotion — water (solvent) plus ammonium thioglycollate (solute).

SOLUTION STRENGTHS The strength or concentration of solutions may be measured in a number of ways:

1   Grams (of solute) dissolved in litres (of solvent), e.g. 1g/litre means one gram dissolved in one litre.

2   A percentage (%) strength gives the number of parts of solute dissolved in 100 parts of solution, e.g. 15% contains 15 parts solute in 100 parts solution. To make a 15% solution, dissolve 15 parts of solute in 85 parts of solvent.

3   The volume strength of a solution is the number of cm^3 (cubic centimetres) of gas produced from 1 cm^3 of the solution. This is a way of measuring the strength of a solution which produces a gas.

Solution strengths can also be measured using relative density (see page 54).

The strength of solution will often help to determine how quickly and effectively a chemical reaction will occur. For example, a strong hydrogen peroxide solution (e.g. 30 vol.) will bleach the hair quicker and more effectively than a weak solution (e.g. 10 vol.).

Emulsions

An emulsion is a suspension of two liquids which will not normally mix, i.e. one will not dissolve in another, such as oil and water. The two liquids are shaken together so that one forms tiny droplets within the other. Emulsifying agents such as detergents or waxes, like lanolin or lanette wax, will prevent the two liquids from separating again and thus maintain the emulsion.

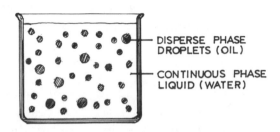

Many emulsions are used by hairdressers, for example, cream shampoo, barrier cream, hand, face and body creams and lotions.

MEASUREMENT

In order to use or prepare many of the solutions and products used in hairdressing you will need to be able to measure them accurately.

Mass

The mass of a substance is equal to its weight (assuming you are on the planet earth!) and can be measured on scales or on a balance. Mass is measured in kilograms (kg).

    1000 grams (g)   =   1kg
    1000 milligrams (mg)   = 1g

Some hair tints are weighed out in grams.

Volume

The volume of a substance is how much space it takes up. Volumes of liquids can be measured in measuring jugs, measuring cylinders, syringes and pipettes. Volumes are measured in cubic metres (m^3) or litres (l).

    1 dm^3 (cubic decimetre)   =   1l (litre)
    1000 cm^3 or cc (cubic centimetres)   =   1l (litre)
    1000 ml (millilitres)   =   1l (litre)
        1ml   =   1cm^3
    10 dl (decilitres)   =   1l (litre)
    100 cl (centilitres)   =   1l (litre)
    1 fl. oz (fluid ounce)   =   30 ml

Reading Liquid Measurements

Pour the product carefully into the measure which should be on a level shelf, then bend down with your eyes level to the product in the measure to read it correctly.

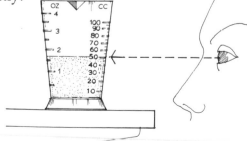

Density

The density of a substance is its mass per unit volume.

$$\frac{mass\ (kg)}{volume\ (m^3)} = \text{density kg/m}^3$$

The density of water is $1g/cm^3$. This means that one gram of water takes up one cubic centimeter of space.

RELATIVE DENSITY This is the density of a substance as compared to the density of water ($1g/cm^3$). Substances which are less dense than water will float on water and have a relative density less than one, e.g. ethanol (alcohol) has a density of 0.79g) cm^3 and a relative density of 0.79.

Substances which are more dense than water will sink and have a relative density greater than one e.g. carbon tetrachloride has a density of $1.6g/cm^3$ and a relative density of 1.6. The relative density of solutions can be measured using a **hydrometer** to give an indication of the solution concentration. A special type of hydrometer known as a **peroxometer** is used to measure the strength of hydrogen peroxide solutions (see Chapter 12 p. 228).

Humidity

Humidity (how much water vapour is present in the air) is measured in units known as percentage (%) relative humidity and is measured by an instrument called a **hygrometer** (see page 57 and 103).

Temperature

Temperature is measured in degrees centigrade (^0C) by a **thermometer** (see page 56).

Time

Time is measured in seconds (s), minutes (min) and hours (hrs) by a clock.

CLEANING IN THE SALON

General salon cleaning

Floors and walls should be washed regularly with hot, soapy water. After drying they should be wiped with antiseptic.

Basins, trolleys and worktops should be cleaned with proprietary (household) cleaning agents according to the manufacturer's instructions.

Mirrors can be cleaned with methylated spirits to remove hairspray, and must be smear-free.

All hairdressing equipment must be thoroughly cleaned and *sterilized* between each client (see page 16).

Laundry

All gowns and towels must be correctly stored and cleaned between each client. There are local by-laws which control this.

IN SALON LAUNDERING Salons may have their own laundry facilities with a good sized washing machine and tumble dryer.

LAUNDERETTES These need to be close by the salon for convenience. If the launderette does not have an attendant, then a member of staff may need to be absent from the salon during washing and drying time.

LAUNDRIES Some laundries own the towels and gowns and hire them out, running a delivery service to the salons.

Other salons may carry a large stock of them to be laundered by a linen company, but a careful check must be made on the amounts being despatched and received.

Heat and Ventilation in the Salon

The temperature of the salon should be warm enough so that clients with wet hair do not feel cold, but not so warm as to be uncomfortable. A temperature of about 20°C is ideal. The salon may be heated by a variety of appliances which may be fixed or portable or part of a central heating system. Whatever the type of heater, heat will flow from the hotter to the cooler surroundings by one or more of the following heat transfer methods:

1 **Conduction** is the transfer of heat from a hotter to a colder material. Heat travels through solids in this way and may be passed by conduction onto other solid objects providing they are touching. Some solids are poor conductors of heat and are called **insulators,** e.g. hair, fat (used as insulators in the body), polystyrene, glass fibre, wood, etc. The best conductors are metals.

2 **Convection** is where heat travels through gases such as air, and through liquids such as water. Hot air or water will rise, cold air and water will sink. By heating the cool air and water a circulation can be achieved. This is called a convection current.

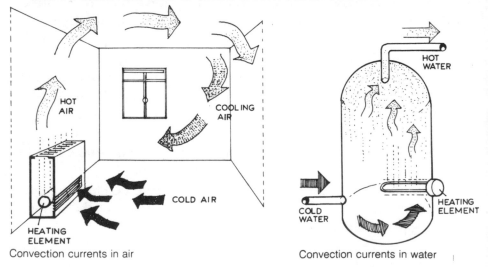

Convection currents in air   Convection currents in water

3 **Radiation** is the transmission of heat in the form of rays, through gasses or space. This heat may be absorbed by objects in the path of the rays enabling them to become hot, but it will not heat the air. Objects may also reflect the rays. Light shiny objects tend to reflect the rays of radiant heat (and remain cool), while dark and dull objects tend to absorb the radiant heat (and become hot).

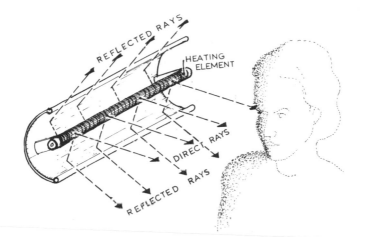

Ventilation

Adequate ventilation in a salon is required for the following reasons:

1   In order to prevent the salon becoming too hot. The temperature of the salon during the day will tend to rise because of heat given off by dryers, hot water and people.

2   To stop the salon becoming too humid. Humidity (water vapour in the air) will also tend to rise during the day because of the evaporation of water from drying hair, wet towels, basins, etc. A humid atmosphere feels uncomfortable and can lead to fatigue. High humidity can also affect the ability of the hair to remain 'set' (see page 102).

3   To ensure a good supply of fresh air. People breathing in a salon will produce stale air with a higher concentration of carbon dioxide (CO_2), as will the burning of fuels like gas and oil. This high CO_2 level may make people feel irritable. The stale air will also contain fumes from solutions such as perm lotions, bleaches, setting lotions and lacquers; as well as germs spread by droplet infection, such as colds and flu (see page 12).

Good ventilation should ensure a supply of fresh air without causing draughts. Natural ventilation includes the use of windows, doors, ventilating bricks, etc. Artificial ventilation involves the use of fans or air conditioning units.

CUSTOMER RELATIONS

Appointments

The receptionist has a key role to play in the salon. Her attitude, appearance and communication skills, including the ability to converse effectively on the telephone, reflect the standards of the salon.

Appointments must be correctly recorded and checked for the right time, date, stylist and service, in the appointment book.

An appointment card is given to the client with all these details written on it.

Each hairstylist needs a certain amount of time to work through each service, e.g. permanent waves and bleaches will take longer than a cut and blow dry, so the amount of time allowed for each individual client is very important.

Occasionally, clients will arrive late or early for appointments and must be dealt with politely and accommodated with the least possible inconvenience.

Client records

Records of each client are necessary in order that she may be contacted if, for example, the appointment has to be changed, or for recording information regarding permanent waves, hair colours, conditioning treatments or for special notes (examples of these are found in the relevant chapters).

Computers are being increasingly used in salons. It is essential to ensure that the computer chosen is one capable of handling the range of software required.

General reception duties

Apart from receiving the clients and checking the appointments, the receptionist must make sure that the client is seated comfortably whilst waiting, and that all belongings are kept in a safe place. Clients should be offered refreshment (coffee, tea, etc.) either before or during their hairdressing service, and magazines or hairstyling books if they are waiting.

The gowning up procedure will vary according to the service to be carried out and is important as no chemicals or cut hair should touch the client's clothes. It is the receptionist or a junior member of staff who usually takes the client's coat.

Displays of retail goods to complement services in the salon are sold at reception.

The reception area must be kept tidy and attractive by the good use of colour, lighting, furniture, flowers and various displays (see page 282).

CUSTOMER ACCOUNTS PROCEDURES

Calculating the bill including VAT

Many hairdressing businesses have to charge VAT (Value Added Tax) to the client because they are supplying goods and services. This tax is then paid back to the Government at a later date. Some salons include VAT within the price, while others add up the bill and then add on the VAT afterwards.

Receiving payments

Normally the salon will display a price list near the reception area (see page 282), but some salons include the prices on their appointment cards. Displays of retail products are often individually priced as they are in normal retail shops, such as chemists.

Clients' bills are written on a bill pad or receipt slip, and usually torn off, given to the client and checked by her before payment is made.

Payment may be either in cash (always check to see it is your national currency, mistakes are often made after journeys abroad), or by cheque (the client's signature must always be in ink), credit card or by account. Cash and cheques are kept in the cash register, but credit card vouchers and accounts are often kept separately.

A typical bill would be:

Date ....

Client's Name ....

Stylist's Name ....

Service	Price
Cutting	☐
Blow Drying	☐
Setting	☐
Permanent Waving	☐
Conditioning Treatment	☐
Colouring	☐
Bleaching/Highlighting	☐
Other Services, e.g. Manicure	☐
Retail Products	_____
Total	_____
(If applicable VAT is charged at 15% of the total cost) (+ VAT)	_____
(Final Total)	_____

CASH Always check the amount of cash the client gives you and the amount of change given back. If the bill is very large, then use a calculator to check the amount is totalled correctly.

Make sure you know how to use your salon's cash register beforehand, and if a receipt is issued then hand it to the client.

CHEQUES   If the client is paying by cheque, then make sure it has been completed correctly.

Most cheques are backed by a cheque guarantee card which must have a valid date, and the signature on it must match the signature written on the cheque. The guarantee card and the cheque must also have the same bank name, bank and account number.

When the client has written on the cheque the correct date, the name of the salon (or business name), the amount of money payable (in words and figures), and signed it, then you must write the cheque card number on the back of the cheque, before issuing the receipt.

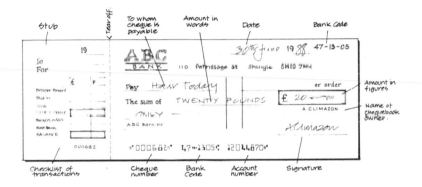

CREDIT CARDS   First check that the credit card is valid, then use the imprinter and correctly complete the voucher, entering the total bill. Check that the client's signature matches the signature on the credit card. Detach the customer's voucher copy, destroy the carbons and safely store the remaining voucher copies.

ACCOUNTS   Client account procedures are settled in accordance with your own salon procedure. Firstly identify the account number, then record the service and ask for the client's signature. Always issue a receipt and correctly file the information.

Occasionally, you may be required by the salon owner/manager to obtain change from the bank for the salon float. This money is kept in the cash register for petty cash (to buy things like coffee or tea) and for giving the clients change.

Make sure you are familiar with banking procedures, as at other times you may be asked to pay in to the bank such things as cash, cheques or credit card vouchers.

MULTIPLE CHOICE QUESTIONS

1 An emulsion is:
  (a) a saturated solution
  (b) a suspension of pigment particles in water
  (c) a suspension of two liquids which will not normally mix
  (d) a solution which releases gas

2 One litre is equal to:
  (a) 10000 cubic centimetres
  (b) 100 cubic centimetres
  (c) 10 centilitres
  (d) 1000 millilitres

3 Which of the following is a 15% solution?
  (a) 1 g of the solute in 25 ml of solution
  (b) 15 g of the solute in 100 ml of solution
  (c) 25 g of the solute in 1 litre of solution
  (d) 25 g of the solute in 250 pints of solution

4 Convection is:
  (a) one way that heat travels through liquids and gases
  (b) a strongly held belief
  (c) the way heat passes through a solid
  (d) a type of radiant heat fire

5 The air in the salon changes during a busy day to become:
  (a) cooler and drier
  (b) warmer and more humid
  (c) saturated and less dense
  (d) stale and less humid

6 A solvent is:
  (a) a type of glue
  (b) a substance which will dissolve in a liquid
  (c) an insoluble substance
  (d) a liquid in which something will dissolve

7 The most suitable temperature for a salon is approximately:
  (a) 65°C   (c) 20°C
  (b) 70°C   (d) 30°C

8 The term 'relative humidity' is used to describe:
  (a) the average level of humidity in salons
  (b) the amount of water vapour in the atmosphere
  (c) extra water vapour in the air
  (d) condensation on walls and windows

9 Which of the following cleaning agents is used to remove hairspray from mirrors?
 (a) methylated spirit
 (b) an antiseptic
 (c) an abrasive powder
 (d) cold salty water

10 Which of the following images would you obtain when using a concave mirror?
 (a) magnified (bigger)
 (b) diminished (smaller)
 (c) back to front
 (d) upside down

11 Infra-red lamps may be used:
 (a) to slow down chemical processes
 (b) to sterilize hairdressing tools
 (c) to apply moist heat
 (d) for 'natural' drying of hair

5

ANALYSIS OF HAIR, SCALP AND SKIN CONDITION

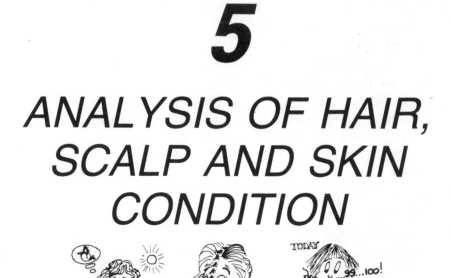

ASSESSING THE CLIENT'S NEEDS

Time in the salon is always a problem. There is never enough of it!

But time spent analyzing the client's hair, scalp and skin condition will enable the hairdresser to give the correct treatment (e.g. cut and blow dry, perm, tint, highlights) for that particular client.

Each individual client needs those products which will suit his or her particular needs, e.g. after a holiday hair condition is often much drier than normal. Analysis will save time and, therefore, money, and the client is more likely to return to your salon another time. Detailed records should be kept (see pages 127, 154, 173, 193, 202 for other types of record cards).

ANALYSIS RECORD CARD

Name: ....

Address: ....

....

Tel. no. (Daytime) ....

Stylist Name: ....

Service Offered

Cutting	Perming
Setting/dressing	Straightening
Blow drying	Colouring
Conditioning treatment	Bleaching/highlights
Other	

Products sold

	During the service	Retail sale
Setting aid		
Dressing aid		
Conditioning		
Perming/straightening		
Colouring/bleaching		
Sundries		

Face shape ....

Special notes ....

Hair density ....

Hair texture ....

Hair condition ....

Hair growth pattern ....

Life-style ....

Special occasion ....

Approximate age ....

Cost of service: ....

Discussion with the client

The hairdresser must disentangle the hair before any hairdressing processes are carried out. This is normally done by brushing which relaxes the client and gives time for discussion (called professionally 'client consultation'). This is the ideal time to look discreetly for any **contra-indications.** A contra-indication is when **not** to continue with the hairdressing process (see Chapter 2 for details). For example:

1 Infestations of the hair or skin by parasites, e.g. lice, itch mites (scabies). The client should be tactfully referred to a medical practitioner.
2 · Infection by highly contagious micro-organisms, e.g. impetigo, ringworm. Again, tactfully refer the client to a medical practitioner.
3 Cuts, abrasions, inflammation which might be subject to secondary infection or further inflammation as a result of hairdressing treatments. Advise the client to return when the condition has healed.

Always discuss the client's general health as her/his state of health will be reflected in the condition of the hair. 'How have you been, lately?' is a question which suggests concern without being over inquisitive.

Certain hair conditions such as natural dryness of the hair and scalp may be corrected by a series of corrective (conditioning) treatments.

Other problems such as excessively porous hair which has been damaged by chemical over-processing may make the hair so stretchy that it will break off if further chemicals are used (see page 152, 222).

Gowning up

A client's clothing must always be adequately protected according to whichever service (cutting, perming, hair colouring, bleaching, conditioning) has been booked (see page 58).

THE STRUCTURE AND CHARACTERISTICS OF THE SCALP AND SKIN

A deeper knowledge of the scalp and skin is necessary for the understanding of all hairdressing processes. Clients today are well educated through the media (TV and magazines) about looking after their hair, and to sell your products sound technical knowledge is necessary,

Structure of the skin

The skin is divided into two layers. The outer layer, the **epidermis** (the germinative layer forms the lowest part of the epidermis) and the inner layer, the **dermis.**

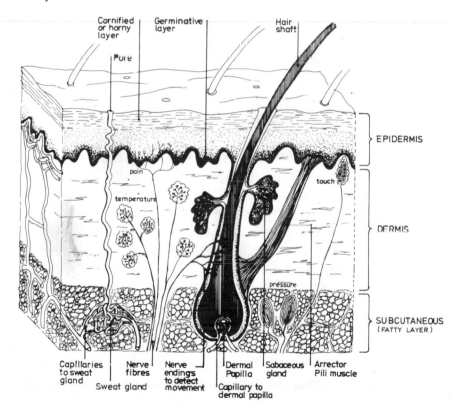

ARRECTOR PILI MUSCLE These can cause the hair to stand erect in animals (and make a goose pimple appear on the skin in man) as a reaction to fear or cold, or to lie flat against the skin in warm conditions.

SEBACEOUS GLANDS These produce a natural oil called **sebum.** This helps to protect the hair, and reflection of light by the oil increases lustre. Underactive sebaceous glands (lack of natural oil) can cause a dry hair and scalp condition. This can be exaggerated by excessive chemical processing (e.g. perming, bleaching, tinting) or exposure to harsh weather conditions (e.g. sun, wind, sea water etc.). Overactive sebaceous glands will produce oiliness of the hair and scalp (greasy hair).

CAPILLARIES These transport blood to and from the skin to provide it with food and oxygen and to remove waste. They also bring the raw materials (nutrients) for hair growth to the dermal papilla.

Characteristics of the scalp and skin and non-infectious scalp conditions

DRYNESS/OILINESS The dryness or oiliness of the skin is due to the amount of sebum produced by Sebaceous glands. Overactivity (Seborrhoea) leads to lank, greasy hair, and areas of greasy skin and may be associated with acne. Sometimes a sebaceous cyst (wen) may form. This occurs if a sebaceous gland becomes blocked.

DANDRUFF (*PITYRIASIS SIMPLEX*) Dry white scales caused by excess shedding skin accumulate on the scalp and may cause considerable itching. Dandruff is not caused by an infection, although micro-organisms such as yeast and bacteria may thrive on the dandruff. Medicated shampoos containing cetrimide or other antiseptics such as hexachlorophene will control the micro-organisms but will not cure dandruff. Anti-dandruff shampoos containing selenium sulphide or zinc pyrithione will reduce cell division in the epidermis and thus reduce dandruff.

PSORIASIS With Psoriasis thick patches of silvery scales are found on the scalp or on the rest of the body. Under the scales the skin may be red and bleeding may occur if scales are removed. A tendency for psoriasis is inherited and attacks may recur, particularly in times of stress. Psoriasis is not infectious and normal hairdressing treatments may be carried out.

HYPERSENSITIVITY OR ALLERGY This can be defined as an abnormal reaction of the body tissues of an individual to a substance which does not affect the majority of people, e.g. certain drugs taken internally, inhaled pollen (hay fever), or skin contact (contact dermatitis).

Contact Dermatitis (or eczema) is an inflammation of the skin which may result in redness, itching, cracking and swelling, caused by a reaction to a particular chemical, e.g. shampoos, permanent wave lotions or tints (para-dyes). hairdressers should wear rubber gloves to avoid this and clients must be given a skin test before tinting, as a precaution against contact dermatitis.

THE STRUCTURE AND CHARACTERISTICS OF HAIR

Structure of hair

The hair shaft is a completely dead structure composed of a protein called **Keratin** which contains the elements carbon, hydrogen, oxygen, nitrogen and sulphur. Like all proteins, keratin is made up of **amino acid units** which are chemically bound together by **peptide linkages** to form long chains known as **polypeptides.** Each hair is composed of three layers, the cuticle, cortex and medulla.

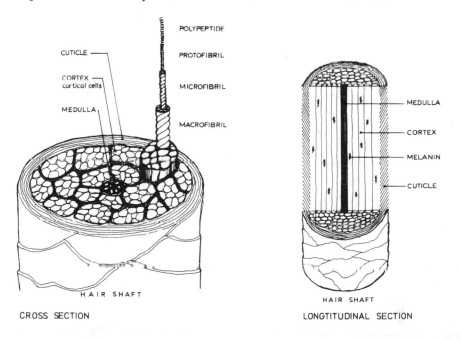

CROSS SECTION   LONGTITUDINAL SECTION

CUTICLE   This consists of 7-10 layers of overlapping scales of keratin which are translucent (only a proportion of the available light passes through — like grease-proof paper). The outer cuticle is tough and holds the whole hair together but may be damaged by chemicals or harsh treatment.

MEDULLA   This is not present in all scalp hairs, particularly if the hair is fine.

CORTEX   The cortex forms the main bulk of the hair. It consists of a system of parallel strands or fibres which are closely bound together by a cementing material (there are some airspaces between them). This gives the hair its strength. Each fibre encloses even finer fibrils. The smallest fibrils are polypeptide chains which have a spiral shape, rather like coiled springs, held together by cross-linkages in a ladder-like structure. These cross-linkages or bonds may be **temporary bonds** (easily broken), i.e. salt linkages and hydrogen bonds. These are important because they affect the elasticity of the hair enabling it to stretch and to spring back when released.

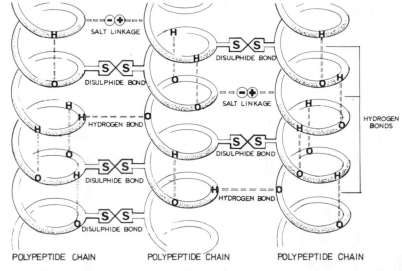

The structure of Keratin

These cross-linkages may also be **permanent bonds** (difficult to break), i.e. disulphide bonds, which are broken and reformed during permanent waving, (see page 170).

The cortex also contains granules of the pigment melanin (brown) and pheomelanin (yellow-red) which are responsible for the colour of hair (see page 199).

Hair Growth

Hair grows by multiplication of cells at the base of the hair follicles in the skin dermis. The follicle undergoes alternate periods of activity and rest. Individual follicles enter the resting stage at different times so that replacement of hair takes place gradually and there is a constant daily loss of about 50-100 scalp hairs.

The average rate of hair growth is 1.25 cm per month. This keeps hairdressers in business! Clients continually need cutting, perming and colouring services.

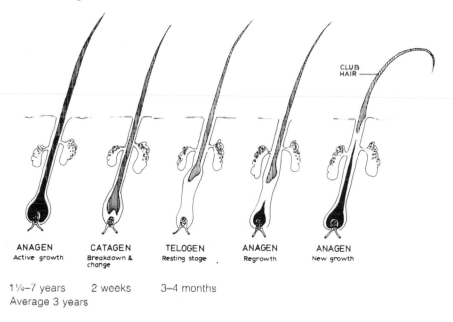

ANAGEN	CATAGEN	TELOGEN	ANAGEN	ANAGEN
Active growth	Breakdown & change	Resting stage	Regrowth	New growth

1¼–7 years	2 weeks	3–4 months		
Average 3 years				

Therefore, some people can grow very long hair, but other people's hair will only grow to shoulder length. It all depends on the length of time of an individual's hair life-cycle.

Characteristics of scalp hair

TYPE OF HAIR   There are three main racial differences in the shape of hair in cross-section:

1   European hair (Caucasian) is oval in shape.
2   Asian hair (Mongoloid) is round in shape.
3   Negroid hair (very curly) is flattened in shape.

HEREDITARY INFLUENCES   Some characteristics affecting hair are passed on from one generation to another. These include hair colour, period length of anagen, catagen and telogen, the amount of curl or wave movement and the tendency for baldness and premature greying. Hair will always grow according to its heredity regardless of chemical or physical treatments.

TYPES OF HAIR GROWTH   Hair grows all over the body except on the lips, palms of the hands and soles of the feet. Fine body hair is called **vellus hair.** Although some of this is found on the scalp, most scalp hair is stronger and more coarse and is called **terminal hair** (which includes long scalp hair, eyebrows, eye lashes, beards and moustaches). A third type of hair, **lanugo hair,** is found on human foetuses and is even finer than vellus hair. All hairs emerge from the surface of the skin.

GROWTH PATTERNS, DIRECTION OF FALL OF HAIR   The angle at which the hair follicle lies within the skin will determine the degree of natural lift (i.e. whether the hair stands on end or lies flat) and the direction of growth of the hair. Scalp hairs tend to grow in groups, causing different sections of the hair to lie in different directions. It is important to consider the natural lie of the hair when planning a suitable style for a client.

DISTRIBUTION OF HAIR/HAIR LOSS (*ALOPECIA*)   General thinning of the hair may be due to a number of factors including hormonal changes (e.g. after childbirth, menopause, pituitary and thyroid disorders), illnesses (e.g. diabetes, anaemia, cancer, illnesses involving high fever), dietary deficiency, severe shock or ageing. Baldness or alopecia can also be caused by a number of factors. For example shock or anxiety can cause *alopecia areata* (patchy baldness). Frequent pulling of the hair may cause traction alopecia. Male pattern baldness (androgenic alopecia) is an inherited characteristic.

TEXTURE AND ABUNDANCE   This is the feel of the hair. Is it coarse, medium or fine? Some people have coarse hair but it is sparse (not much of it), others may have fine hair but lots of it (abundant). There are approximately 100,000 hairs growing on the average scalp.

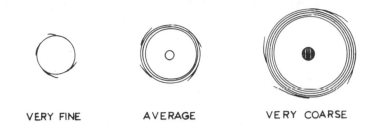

VERY FINE   AVERAGE   VERY COARSE

ELASTICITY   The elasticity of hair is due to the coiled structure of keratin in the cortex. Wet hair stretches more than dry hair. Hair that is severely damaged by chemicals or harsh treatment may lose elasticity. It may be tested with a special machine called a tensile strength meter, or by pulling it between the fingers.

DRYNESS/OILINESS   The amount of sebum produced by the sebaceous glands will partially determine this. Damaged hair will tend to be dry, particularly at the ends (points).

POROSITY   Hair is said to be porous because it can absorb liquids into the cortex. The porosity depends on the state of the cuticle. If the scales are damaged or opened by heat or chemical action (such as alkalis) or by exposure to harsh weather conditions (such as sun, wind, rain, etc.) porosity is increased. Substances such as sebum, hair lacquer and conditioning lotions will decrease porosity. Hair is more porous towards the ends (points). All hair is **hygroscopic**, i.e. it absorbs moisture from the air.

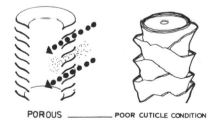

POROUS ————— POOR CUTICLE CONDITION

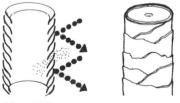

RESISTANT ————— GOOD CUTICLE CONDITION

Hair porosity

SPLIT ENDS/HAIR BREAKAGE   The hair shaft may be damaged mechanically by severe backcombing, ponytails, plaiting and by the use of spiked or excessively tight rollers. Chemical damage may result from the use of alkaline products, too strong perm lotion or bleaches. This damage will often result in hair breakage, such as split ends (*Fragilatis crinium*) and *Trichorrhexis nodosa* where the hair breaks off at small split swellings in the hair shaft.

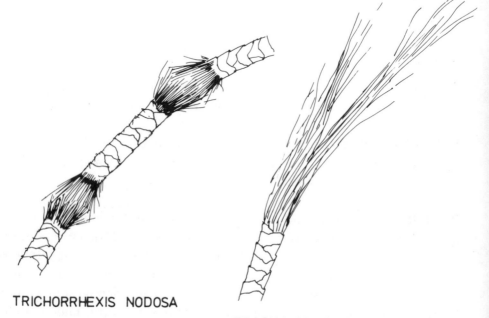

TRICHORRHEXIS NODOSA

FRAGILITAS CRINIUM

COLOUR   The natural colour of the hair is an inherited characteristic due mainly to pigments within the cortex of the hair — melanin (brown) and pheomelanin (yellow-red) and Trichosiderin (red). The natural colour may be made lighter by bleaching, or extra colour may be added to the natural colour during the process of tinting. In some cases the two processes may be carried out together and the hair may be dyed lighter than the natural shade. Any of these treatments may cause damage to the hair.

Greying of hair is the progressive loss of colour known as **canites** (pronounced 'Kanishiez'). 'Grey hair' is a mixture of white and coloured hairs and is usually due to a combination of age and hereditary factors but may also be caused by ill health or nervous conditions.

LUSTRE   Hair which is in good condition has lustre (shiny surface). This is because hair with a smooth surface and a thin coating of sebum, reflects light evenly and in one direction only. Hair which has a rough surface, because the cuticle is in poor condition due to chemical or mechanical damage, or which has too much or too little sebum coating it, will lack lustre. This hair will appear dull because light is not reflected evenly from it but diffused in all directions.

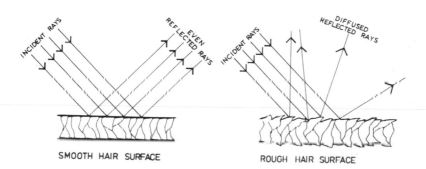

SMOOTH HAIR SURFACE   ROUGH HAIR SURFACE

CURL   Hair may be naturally curly or curls may be produced by artificial means such as blow-drying or setting the hair (temporary) or by permanent waving.

Sometimes it is difficult to tell if the hair is naturally curly or not. When the hair is wet if the curl is even all over then it is possibly permanently waved.

ANALYSIS OUTCOME

Consider all the information in this chapter. Should the service now proceed? If so, which service? Could the client benefit from a conditioning treatment, a permanent wave or a hair-colour? If there are any contra-indications, tactfully advise medical referral, and the client will be sure to come back to you — the caring hairdresser.

MULTIPLE CHOICE QUESTIONS

1 A contra-indication is:
   (a)   a type of diffuse alopecia
   (b)   an infestation by animal parasites
   (c)   a fungal infection
   (d)   when a hairdressing process should not be carried out
2 Canites is a term used to describe:
   (a)   the greying of hair
   (b)   the abundance of hair
   (c)   the porosity of hair
   (d)   the elasticity of hair
3 The period of active hair growth is known as:
   (a)   telogen
   (b)   catagen
   (c)   alopecia
   (d)   anagen
4 The type of hair which grows on the scalp is known as:
   (a)   terminal hair
   (b)   lanugo hair
   (c)   vellus hair
   (d)   coarse hair
5 The sebaceous glands produce:
   (a)   sweat
   (b)   sebum
   (c)   epidermal scales
   (d)   semen
6 Dandruff is sometimes known as:
   (a)   psoriasis
   (b)   eczema
   (c)   Fragilatis
   (d)   Pityriasis
7 Nourishment for the growing hair is supplied by the:
   (a)   blood capillaries
   (b)   sweat glands
   (c)   sebaceous glands
   (d)   epidermal layer
8 The natural colour pigments of the hair are found:
   (a)   in between the cuticle scales
   (b)   throughout the cortex layer

   (c)   throughout the medulla layer
   (d)   on the cuticle scale

9 Hair is made from a substance called:
   (a)   keratin
   (b)   melanin
   (c)   sebum
   (d)   pheomelanin

10 Many hairdressing processes cause chemical changes in:
   (a)   the cortex
   (b)   the medulla
   (c)   the cuticle
   (d)   the dermis

11 Substances which allow some, but not all, of the available light to
pass through them are known as:
   (a)   opaque
   (b)   transparent
   (c)   translucent
   (d)   incandescent

12 The spiral-shaped fibrils in keratin molecules are:
   (a)   polypeptides
   (b)   amino acids
   (c)   di-sulphide bonds
   (d)   polyvinyls

13 The outermost layer of the skin is the:
   (a)   dermis
   (b)   subcutaneous fatty layer
   (c)   basal layer
   (d)   epidermis

14 The daily loss of scalp hair is approximately:
   (a)   80-100
   (b)   2-10
   (c)   200-250
   (d)   250-300

15 Psoriasis is:
   (a)   a non-infectious condition
   (b)   an infestation
   (c)   a bacterial infection
   (d)   a viral disease

6
SHAMPOOING

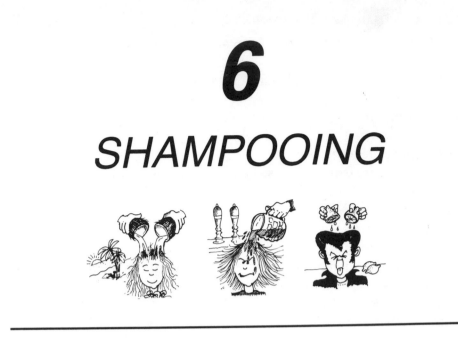

One of the first procedures learned in the salon is shampooing a client's hair. The client is paying for this service so it must be done properly, and better than he or she could do at home!

Clean hair is a great morale booster, and a thorough shampoo will remove all the dirt, grease, epithelial debris (extra flakes of dead skin), hair lacquer or spray, setting aids and mousse and even temporary colours (coloured mousse or gel).

Shampooing is always necessary before perming hair as excess hairspray or mousse will stop the perm lotion from working. When clients have tints, bleaches or highlights they have to be removed by thorough shampooing to stop them continuing to colour or bleach the hair.

Children, old people, the handicapped and the disabled may need special care and attention, as careless shampooing may worry them about further procedures.

There are two methods of shampooing

↙   ↘

Wet Methods   *Dry Methods*

) soapless detergents   spirit/alcohol
water +) soapless detergents + additives   powder
) soap

Usually done at the basin   Usually done at the
                                                dressing position

Hard and soft water

Water is a good solvent and many different substances dissolve in it. Some of the dissolved impurities in tap water (i.e. calcium and magnesium salts) make it hard. Hardness in water causes the formation of scum (calcium stearate) when soap is used but not when soapless detergents are applied. Soaps will not lather when added to hard water, although soapless detergents will. In addition hard water causes 'furring' in steamers, pipes (especially hot pipes), shower roseheads, etc. Distilled or deionized water has been treated to remove impurities, including those which cause hardness. This 'soft water' is therefore suitable for steamers, shower roseheads and the salon water supply.

   Two types of hardness exist:

1 **Temporary hardness** which is caused by **calcium or magnesium bicarbonates.** This type of hardness can be removed by boiling or by water softeners.
2 **Permanent hardness** which is caused by **calcium** or **magnesium sulphates.** This type of hardness is removed only by water softeners, e.g. sodium ion-exchange resins and sodium hexametaphosphate (Calgon).

Detergency

By itself water is not a good cleansing agent. A detergent (or **surfactant**) is a substance which acts with water to make things clean. Its action involves three stages.

1 Detergents act as wetting agents

Water has high surface tension which has the effect of producing a 'skin' on the surface of the water, thus preventing the water from spreading easily over surfaces like hair and fabrics.

When added to water, detergents will lower the surface tension and make water droplets flatten out, so 'wetting' the surface.

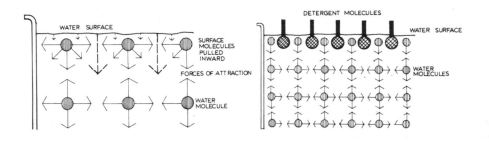

Surface tension in water   Detergent molecules in water reduce surface tension

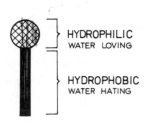

A detergent molecule

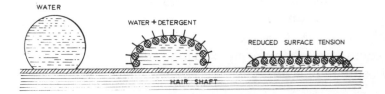

High surface tension   Low surface tension

2 Detergents act as emulsifying agents

Detergents attach themselves to greasy (fatty) dirt and thereby remove it from the hair. The detergent molecules surround the greasy dirt and hold it in suspension within the water, i.e. the detergent produces an emulsion (an emulsion consists of minute droplets of one liquid suspended in another (see page 52).

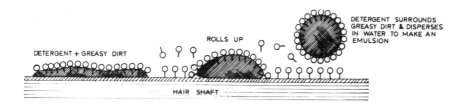

Detergents act with water to remove grease and dirt

3 Detergents coat hair and dirt

The detergent molecules repel one another, so the dirt will not resettle on the hair.

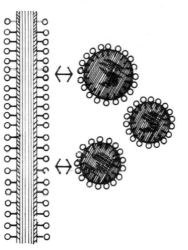

Dirt will not resettle

TYPES OF DETERGENTS

SOAP Soaps such as **sodium stearate** (hard soap) and **potassium stearate** (soft soap) will act as detergents. They are rarely used in shampoos since they form a scum of calcium stearate with hard water. This scum is left in the basin after washing your hands — imagine that left in your hair! Soaps are alkaline in solution (pH 8–9) causing roughening of the hair cuticle (see page 153).

SOAPLESS DETERGENTS The **lauryl sulphates** are usually used in soapless shampoos, e.g. **sodium lauryl ether sulphate, triethanolamine lauryl sulphate.** They are manufactured from vegetable oils by treating them with sulphuric acids. They are neutral (ph7) so leave the hair cuticle smooth (see Chapter 9 page 153).

DRY SHAMPOOING Sometimes it is impossible to wash the client's hair, for instance if there is no hot water (from a power cut), or if the client has a tender scalp after illness. Then the hair can be dry cleaned (like clothes) by the use of the following:

1 **Spirit/alcohol**
   Solvents such as white spirit (petroleum liquid) and trichloroethylene may be used as wig-cleaners. However, these solvents are highly inflammable or highly toxic and are not therefore used on clients.

2 **Dry powders**
   These consist of an alkaline substance (e.g. borax or washing soda) together with an absorbent powder (e.g. talc, Fullers Earth, French chalk). They absorb grease when brushed through the hair but it is difficult to remove all traces of powder, and they can therefore leave the hair looking dull. They are rarely used in salon work.

METHODS

Preparation

CONTRA-INDICATIONS TO SHAMPOOING During the analysis of hair, scalp and skin condition, any infestations (such as head lice), scalp cuts, abrasions or infections would have been noticed. (Remember the word contra-indication means when not to do something.)

CLIENT COMFORT   There are various types of washbasins used in salons, e.g.

> Front wash
> Back wash
> Side wash

Clients may ask for a particular type of washbasin according to their needs. Tall or short clients, children, or people with back problems often have difficulties with certain shaped washbasins and different backwash chair types.

Most backwash chairs are especially sprung so that when the client leans backwards the back of the chair reclines and she can comfortably be positioned. Frontwash basins are more difficult to use, and the client's face must be protected, particularly from dangerous chemicals being used near the eyes (e.g. removing tints after processing). A small hand towel (covered with paper tissue to collect any excess make-up, if necessary) should be offered to the client as a face protection. Remember the client should feel comfortable and relaxed after shampooing — check to make sure.

PROTECTIVE CLOTHING   Clean protective clothing must always be used. Clients need a lot of care during shampooing and there are many ways of gowning up. Gowns or aprons, shampoo capes and towels are placed around the client after the client consultation. These should be secure but must not restrict the client's neck movements.

BRUSHING AND COMBING   Hair must be thoroughly disentangled before shampooing. Open tufted brushes which penetrate the hair, or wide toothed combs can improve client comfort. Usually hair is brushed first, then combed to double check that it is tangle free.

Brushing is important not only for disentanglement, but to help remove dirt, dust, excess dandruff and hairspray before starting. It is a good time to check the hair and scalp for any contra-indications to shampooing, without it being obvious to the client.

Good brushing will stimulate the sebaceous glands to produce sebum (natural hair grease) and spread it along the hair shaft.

Brushing and combing can be extremely uncomfortable for the client if it is not carried out correctly. You should start brushing from the points or ends of the hair, holding the middle lengths of the hair firmly if it is long. Always work from the nape area (back) first, then taking 40 mm sections, carefully work towards the front. This should be done several times before combing the hair through.

Two brushes can be used, holding one in each hand, and this is called double brushing. Brushes must always be held correctly, that is with the first finger and thumb well down the handle and with the other fingers encircling it to allow good, flexible wrist movements. Brushing hair is an excellent exercise to loosen the wrists. All hairdressers work better if their wrists are both supple and flexible.

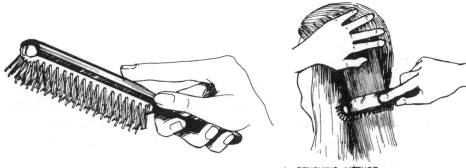

a. BRUSH HOLD   b. BRUSHING METHOD

Both brushes and combs must have rounded teeth or bristles, as sharp edges can catch the client's scalp and cause cuts, abrasions and inflammation. They must be cleaned after each use by removing loose hairs, immersing in hot soapy water, rinsing in cold water, drying thoroughly and then sterilizing.

Types of shampoo

The organized hairdresser will always decide which type of shampoo (and conditioner if applicable) is best suited to the client's hair and scalp conditions and gather these materials beforehand. If there are two problems, e.g. dandruff and dry hair, then deal with the worst problem first and suggest further treatments for the other.

SHAMPOOS Shampoos usually consist of a mixture of water and soapless detergent. They may contain additives such as:

1 Medicating agents to control bacteria or infestation, e.g. coal tar, cetrimide, hexachlorophene and malathion.
2 Conditioners to improve the hair's condition and to help control static electricity, e.g. lanolin, lemon, egg, beer.

3 Anti-dandruff agents such as zinc pyrithione and selenium sulphide.

The following table is a general guide relating hair and scalp conditions to suitable shampoos.

Conditions	Shampoo type
Dry hair (Permed/tinted/ bleached, i.e. chemically treated)	Almond/coconut, lanolin, egg
Flyaway hair	Beer
Scalps with dandruff	Medicated and anti-dandruff (Selenium sulphide or zinc pyrithione) N.B. This will increase dryness
Greasy hair	Plain lemon or soapless — clear liquid. N.B. Soapless is used before perming or dry shampoos — liquid/powder
Very dry hair	Conditioning shampoo
Hair with excessive hairspray	Shampoo with lacquer-removing solvent

Always read any manufacturer's instructions, as some shampoos may need to be left on the hair for several minutes, whilst others can be rinsed out immediately.

Occasionally, only one shampoo need be given instead of two, but again check all instructions.

It is very important not to waste shampoo, and some have thicker consistencies than others. Always check to see if the shampoo product needs to be diluted before use.

Water temperatures

Using the water spray during shampooing takes practice, so test the controls first. Both water sprays and mixing valves need regular maintenance because of lime scale deposits ('furring up') from hard water. This can cause blockages and less water pressure to be available making rinsing the hair take a long time. Look at the rose and spray heads regularly to see if they need cleaning.

The temperature of the water should be as warm as the client can comfortably stand. *Do not* forget to ask her. Generally, cooler water is used after harsh chemical treatments such as tinting or bleaching when the scalp is more sensitive.

Test the temperature of the water by spraying it either on your wrist or the back of your hand, and adjust it as necessary. Turn the cold tap on first at a moderate rate of flow, and then mix in water from the hot tap until the correct temperature is reached. *Remember* that the sensitivity of the scalp to temperature will vary from person to person, and that what is comfortably warm to one person may be too hot for another. Adjust accordingly for each individual client.

Shampooing

WETTING THE HAIR   Once the water temperature has been adjusted to suit the client the hair must be wetted thoroughly. The water spray must be held close to the head and directed away from the face following the different angles of the head shape.

Start at the centre of the forehead, making a barrier with your free hand to protect the client's face from water. Sweep the water over the hair using the spray and hand together. Cup the hand when above and around the ears, patting the water up into the nape hair. Remember to hold the spray until the water is turned off!

APPLYING THE SHAMPOO   To avoid the hair becoming fly-away or unmanageable look at the length and thickness of the hair and use the correct type and amount of shampoo. Use less shampoo for less hair, to avoid wastage and making the hair too fluffy and uncontrollable.

The shampoo must then be applied in several places over the hair a little at a time. Do not apply shampoo directly on to the head, but run it first over the back of your hand and then onto the head.

This will prevent the shock of cold shampoo on the head. Use your hands flat to spread the shampoo through the hair. Always apply shampoo carefully without missing any areas and avoid allowing any to enter the client's ears or eyes as both can be very sensitive.

MASSAGE   Starting at the centre of the forehead by the hairline, push your fingers through the hair to the scalp and begin to massage with the pads of your fingers (not your fingernails).

Do not keep your palms flat, but arch your palms and fingers as though you were grasping a large ball. Open and close the whole hand, whilst keeping the fingers well spread, and allow the fingers of one hand to pass between those of the other.

When the shampoo is being stroked onto the hair, it is called an **effleurage** massage movement, whereas the more circular massage is known as a **rotary** movement. Some clients enjoy a really deep massage, which is similar to a rotary movement, but kneads the scalp, this is called a **petrissage** movement.

All scalp massage has a beneficial effect in that the blood flow is stimulated to the dermis (the skin) and nutrients will reach the hair bulb to stimulate hair growth.

RINSING   The client will be relaxed after a good massage technique, and the hair must now be rinsed thoroughly to complete the process.

Rinse the hair until the water runs clear and check all around the front and back hairlines to ensure that there is neither shampoo nor conditioner, if used, left, before gently squeezing out any surplus water from the hair.

BRINGING THE CLIENT TO AN UPRIGHT POSITION
There are many personal variations in the method of using shampoo towels, but what is really important is that the client should remain dry and comfortable.

Bring the client to an upright position by asking her to sit up when you are ready.

TOWEL DRYING THE HAIR   It is often better to ask the client to come over to the dressing position with the towel turban wrapped securely around her hair before towel drying thoroughly. This is for safety reasons, so that she can see clearly where she is going.

Preparing the hair for the next procedure

PREPARING THE HAIR   The hair is normally disentangled by using a wide toothed comb in the same manner as brushing, i.e.

working from nape to forehead, points to roots, and holding the mid-lengths of the hair if it is long to avoid any discomfort.

Most hair (except Negroid and very curly Caucasian hair which tends to dry quickly) is then towel dried by gently rubbing or pressing it against a towel. This is to remove excess moisture which may dilute other products, and to reduce the drying time.

Make sure that the towel remaining over the client's shoulders is dry, as it may be left there for some time, and the dampness could seep through to clothing underneath.

Cleaning the work station

The work station is the shampoo area, which includes the washbasin, the backwash chair and the surrounding worktops and floors. Products and equipment must be cleared away and the washbasin cleaned thoroughly. This must include removing any excess hair (which is insoluble and will clog up the drainage systems), any shampoo, tints, bleaches or permanent wave neutralising products left on or around the area, and also regularly disinfecting all surfaces.

MULTIPLE CHOICE QUESTIONS

1 The chemical name for scum is:
  (a) sodium stearate
  (b) potassium stearate
  (c) magnesium carbonate
  (d) calcium stearate

2 Temporary hard water may be caused by:
  (a) calcium sulphate
  (b) magnesium bicarbonate
  (c) magnesium sulphate
  (d) calcium stearate

3 Distilled water is most suitable for steamers because:
  (a) it does not cause 'furring'
  (b) it produces more steam per volume of water
  (c) it does not conduct electricity
  (d) it does not get as hot as tap water

4 A hydrophobic substance is one which:
  (a) loves water
  (b) hates water
  (c) produces a lather with water
  (d) conditions the hair whilst shampooing

5 Boiling permanently hard water will produce:
  (a) soft water   (c) 'furring'
  (b) scum   (d) no change

6 An example of a water softener is:
  (a) sodium hexametaphosphate
  (b) calcium stearate
  (c) sodium lauryl sulphate
  (d) hexachlorophene

7 Soapless detergents with hard water will:
  (a) produce a lather
  (b) produce a scum
  (c) cause 'furring' in pipes
  (d) produce salt water

8 When added to water, detergents will:
  (a) increase surface tension
  (b) coat the surface tension
  (c) lower the surface tension
  (d) wet the surface tension

9 Shampoo containing zinc pyrithione is used to:
   (a) condition the hair
   (b) reduce dandruff
   (c) control bacteria
   (d) kill nits

10 Soapless detergents remove grease by forming:
   (a) a solution
   (b) a suspension
   (c) an emulsion
   (d) an acid

11 Which chemical should be used for cleaning wigs?
   (a) methylated spirits
   (b) ethanol
   (c) trichlorethylene ✓
   (d) sodium stearate

12 Hair should be disentangled by working from:
   (a) nape to forehead; points to roots
   (b) forehead to nape; roots to points
   (c) forehead to nape; points to roots
   (d) nape to forehead; roots to points

13 Beer shampoo is normally used for:
   (a) greasy hair
   (b) dry hair
   (c) fly away hair
   (d) lank hair

14 When removing bleach from the hair the water temperature should be:
   (a) hot
   (b) cold
   (c) very hot
   (d) tepid

15 Shampoo should be applied:
   (a) directly on to the hair at the crown
   (b) to the back of the hand first
   (c) directly on to the hair in various places
   (d) in a line across the crown from ear to ear

7

SETTING AND DRESSING OUT

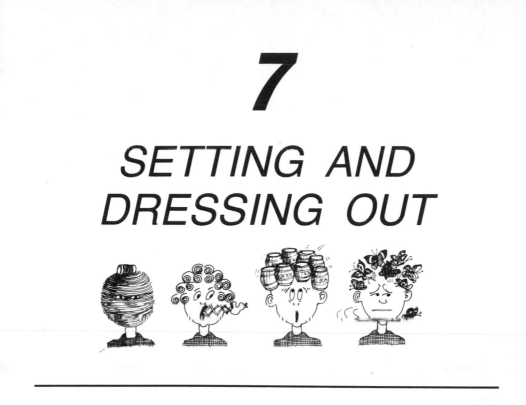

Straight hair may be made curly or wavy by setting, blow drying or finger waving, and curly hair can be made straight by the same methods. Using these techniques wet hair is stretched and then dried in its new position. Dry hair may also be styled by the use of heated styling equipment such as tongs, hot brushes, heated rollers, etc.

PREPARATION

Discussion with the client

First, discuss the client's requirements and remember to ask about any previous treatments that may have been done to the hair, e.g. perms, hair-colours or previous hair styles. If you have styled the client's hair before, still ask questions as you may be able to improve your services.

Hair styles may relate to particular occasions, for example:

1 Everyday styles.
2 Evening styles (and special occasions such as weddings).

3   Fashion styles.
4   Fantasy styles (for hairdressing shows).
5   Historical dressings (often on wigs).

Show the client your style books. Many commercial ones are available, but your own book is more impressive. If you have produced some styles and had them photographed professionally then the client can see your capabilities (see Chapter 15).

Gowning up

See page 45. It is better to gown up after discussion with clients so that not only their clothes and lifestyle are considered but also their height and body shape can be more clearly seen.

HAIR AND SCALP SUITABILITY

You should look carefully at the client's hair and scalp in order to assess the correct treatment and style for her/him.

HAIR (see Chapter 5)   You should consider the following:

1   Hair type — Caucasian, Asian, Negroid, i.e. the amount of natural curl.
2   Texture — coarse, medium or fine.
3   Abundance — the amount of hair.
4   Length — observe the overall length and layers. Remember the weight of naturally curly or wavy long hair keeps it looking long. When it is cut shorter, then styled, it may curl more and appear even shorter than expected!
5   Porosity — how much moisture the hair can absorb.
6   Condition — how dry or greasy the hair is.
7   Growth patterns — the natural growth of the hair (see page 72 and 131).
8   Elasticity — how much the hair can stretch and return to its original length.
9   Previous treatments — refer to the record card regarding perms, colours or treatments and ask the client.

SCALP (see Chapters 2 and 5)   You should consider the following:

1   Excessively dry — flaking skin scales.
2   Inflammation — redness or soreness.
3   Abrasions — if small cover with collodian, if large do not proceed.
4   Cuts — do not proceed unless cuts are suitably covered and protected.

Other considerations

As well as considering the suitability of the hair and scalp, you should also take into account aesthetic considerations, i.e. face shapes, and suitable styles are extremely important (see Chapter 14). This is why some styles suit one person very well, but other styles may look less good on the same person.

The client's life-style, occupation and personality is important. For example:

1   Life style — a young working mother will not have much time to spend on her hair.
2   Occupations — the Police Force and the Nursing professions have strict rules about the length of hair.
3   Personality — introverts will not be as daring with new styles as extroverts. Often clients are worried about other people's reactions to a new hairstyle, and will say 'I'm not sure if my husband/wife will like it'.

The client's age is also important. Sometimes it is difficult to judge how old a person is, but generally softer styles with more movement are flattering on older people.

The health of a person is often reflected in their hair, and people who are unwell often have lank, lifeless hair that is difficult to handle (see Chapter 5).

EQUIPMENT

Back mirrors (hand mirrors)

See page 41. These are usually plane mirrors,

Brushes

See page 47.

Brushes are used both before styling to remove tangles and fine debris and during styling to blow dry or for dressing. They must be regularly cleansed, dried and sterilized **between each client.**

Professional hairdressing brushes are often sold at reception areas to increase profits, so discuss the benefits of each with your client.

FLAT BRUSHES See page 114. This is an all purpose type of brush often made of synthetic materials. They may be open or close tufted. Open tufted brushes penetrate hair meshes more easily, but close tufted brushes are used to give perfectly smooth finishes whilst dressing.

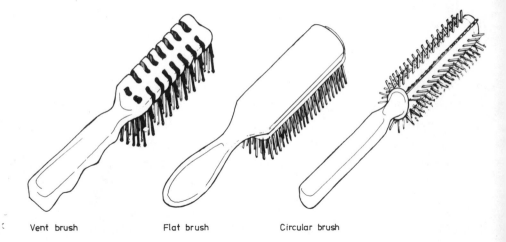

Vent brush   Flat brush   Circular brush

VENT BRUSHES See page 114. These are usually hardwearing and made of synthetic materials. They have open spaces at the back to allow air to flow through during blow drying.

CIRCULAR BRUSHES See page 115. These come in a variety of diameters and are useful for blow drying and styling.

Pins and clips

See page 47. These are used whilst sectioning and securing the hair and during setting, for securing pin curls or rollers. They require regular cleaning and sterilizing after use.

FINE HAIRPINS   These may be used during dressing procedures, often whilst putting hair up. They are not very strong and will only hold small amounts of hair. They are often available in several shades to match the client's hair colour. Sometimes they are used to secure pin curls during setting, as they do not mark the hair as much as metal double pronged clips.

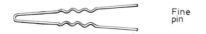

Fine
pin

STRAIGHT PINS   These straight strong pins are made of metal and must **never** be used during chemical processes, as they will discolour the hair. They are available in different lengths and are used to secure rollers during setting and for dressing long hair.

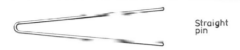

Straight
pin

PLASTIC SETTING PINS   These are not often used in setting because they tend to distort the hair, but they are **safe** to use during perming as they do not react with chemicals.

Setting
pin

GRIPS   Hairgrips are made of metal and are available in a variety of colours to match the client's own. They are normally used whilst dressing longer hair.

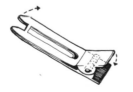

Grip

DOUBLE PRONGED CLIPS   These may be made of metal or plastic and are usually used for securing pin curls.

Double
pronged
clip

SECTIONING CLIPS These are normally made of metal and are used for holding large sections of hair during setting, cutting, perming, straightening, hair-colouring and bleaching.

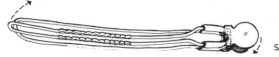

Sectioning clip

BUTTERFLY CLIPS These are used in the same way as sectioning clips but are often made of plastic with 'teeth' to secure the hair more firmly.

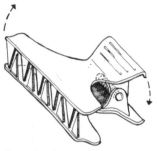

Butterfly clip

Combs

These are only used to remove tangles, but are needed for parting and sectioning as well as dressing hair. They must be kept perfectly clean and sterilized **between every client.**

TAIL COMB This has a plastic tail and usually one size of teeth and is usually used for setting hair.

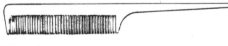

Tail comb

PIN-TAIL COMB This is similar to a tail comb with one size of teeth, but the metal tail is useful for dividing the hair into fine sections during perm winding and weaving out highlights. (In America these are known as rat tail combs.)

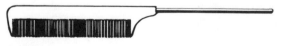

Pin Tail comb

SETTING (DRESSING OR SALON) COMB These have two sizes of teeth and are made in varying lengths and sizes. The larger teeth are useful for disentangling hair.

Straight combs are used for dressing out, cutting, sectioning and finger waving.

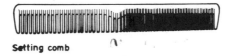

Setting comb

These combs must be held properly to allow maximum wrist movement and flexibility (see Chapter 8).

CUTTING COMB These are similar to, but smaller than, setting combs and are flexible. They are used for very short hair work, often in the nape and sides of a haircut during scissor over comb cutting.

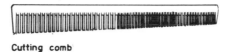

Cutting comb

RAKE These combs sometimes have a handle but always have wide spaced teeth. They are used for disentangling and do not tear and stretch wet hair, so are good for combing products through, such as tints and conditioners.

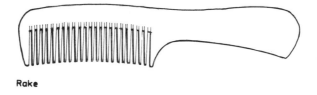

Rake

METAL Metal combs are only used on dry hair because they are not flexible, and would tear and split wet hair. They conduct heat and are good for blow waving.

Sometimes hair is very 'fly-away' during dressing out or during dry cutting and these combs help to reduce static electricity.

AFRO These combs have wide spread teeth and a handle and are used for styling negroid hair, naturally curly European hair or 'natural dry' perms.

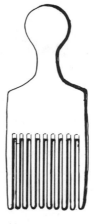

Afro

Dryers

Always learn how to control both the heat and spread settings of all dryers before use.

All dryers contain a **thermostat** which is a device for controlling temperature. It acts by cutting off the electricity supply to a heating element once the selected temperature has been reached. This switches off the heating element and the dryer cools down a little. The thermostat now switches on the heating element again. By switching the heating element on and off in this way, the pre-selected temperature is maintained.

HOOD DRYERS These are used to dry hair after it has been set in 'pli' i.e. where rollers or pin curls have been used, or for natural drying under a slow speed setting. They may be free standing and portable allowing the dryer to be moved to the dressing position, attached to the back of several chairs (a drying bank), or attached to the wall and manoeuvred into position for drying. Always remember to show your client how to use the drier controls (see page 43).

HAND DRYERS AND INFRA-RED DRYERS   See page 43.

Hair nets

Professional hair nets are used to secure the 'pli' whilst the client is under the hood dryer. They are very strong and must be secured properly. If the back of the 'pli' is combed smooth, without rollers and pin curls (often used in competition work), then the net must be secured so that it does not distort the hair whilst drying. Ear shields may be used to protect the ears from hairdryers, but must be sterile. Disposable paper shields are available.

Rollers

Hair rollers are used mainly on wet hair during setting, but may be used on dry hair with setting or dressing aids before combing out (dressing the hair). They are normally secured with straight pins, but some are secured with double pronged clips.

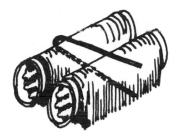

Rollers secured with straight pin

Spiky rollers hold the hair better in place, but are difficult to both clean and remove. Smooth rollers are hard to hold in the hair but give a smoother finish. Different size rollers are available for various effects, they are often colour coded. Generally, the smaller the roller, the tighter the curl. Rollers must be clean and always sterile.

Equipment trolleys

These may be free standing and portable or wall mounted. The free standing trolleys should be placed close to the operator in a safe position and either on the right or the left hand according to whether the operator is right or left handed.

Water sprays

These need regular cleaning as hard water salts often clog up the fine sprays.

They are used to spray water on the hair for more control during wet styling. It is more comfortable for the client if the water is warm.

Sterilizers

See pages 16 and 17.

MATERIALS

Always check the manufacturer's instructions before use.

For use on wet hair

Various setting and styling aids are available and may be in the form of liquids, gels, mousse, gums, oils or creams.

They may be used to make the style longer lasting, to add colour or create different effects (e.g. 'wet look' gels). Some have special additives for dry or greasy hair and many are available in individual containers. Many contain the plastic polyvinyl pyrrolidone (PVP). They help to maintain a set by reducing the amount of water vapour taken up by the hair from the atmosphere (see page 102).

For use on dry hair

Hair sprays or lacquer are used during dressing to control the hair and give more hold and body. They do this in the same way as setting aids by reducing the hygroscopic properties of the hair.

They may be either plastic (PVP) or shellac based.

They are available in aerosol form, but some manufacturers supply refillable containers for economy. Too much hairspray in the atmosphere can be dangerous and so good salon ventilation is essential (see page 57).

DRYING THE HAIR

Hair dries as the water **evaporates** away. The water changes from a liquid (on the hair) to a gas (in the air). This is a physical change (see Chapter 4, page 51).

The rate of evaporation (how quickly the hair dries) will increase:

1   When the temperature rises.
2   When the air surrounding the hair has low humidity.
3   When the air surrounding the hair is kept moving — this moves the water-laden air away from the hair.
4   When a large surface area of hair is exposed to the air. Thus loose hair will dry more quickly than hair wrapped round in a curler.

The aim of hair dryers therefore is to speed up the rate of evaporation by blowing warm air across the hair surface.

As the water evaporates it has a cooling effect on its surroundings. This means that clients with wet hair will tend to feel cool even though you, with dry hair, may feel warm. This cooling effect of evaporation also explains why perfume or after-shave feels cold when it touches the skin. Because these are spirit- (alcohol)- based products, they evaporate quickly and by so doing, cool the skin.

THE EFFECT OF SETTING ON HAIR

Hair setting is a temporary change of the hair shape. Straight hair can be made curly or wavy and curly hair can be made straighter. Setting the hair includes also the techniques of blow styling and heat or dry styling (with electrical equipment such as tongs, hot brushes, crimping irons and heated rollers). Hair may be set because of its elastic and porous nature.

The hair structure is held together by chemical bonds which may be permanent or temporary (see page 70). In hairdressing processes these bonds are broken and reformed. In order to set the hair, the temporary **hydrogen bond** is affected (the permanent bonds are unaffected). Each hydrogen bond is weak but there are very many of them so their combined effect is great.

Cohesive setting (wet setting)

In dry hair the hydrogen bonds limit the amount the hair can stretch since they hold the coils of the polypeptide chains close together. This is known as **alpha (α) keratin.**

When the hair is wet, many of the hydrogen bonds are broken by water, so the hair is able to stretch more. It is while the hair is wet that it is stretched over the curler (or brush as in blow-drying). Hair in this stretched condition is known as **beta (β) keratin.**

As the hair dries, the water evaporates and the hydrogen bonds reform. However, the 'old bonds' are now too far apart to reform so new hydrogen bonds, which hold the hair in the stretched (β keratin) condition are formed. Therefore the curl is maintained even though the curler is removed.

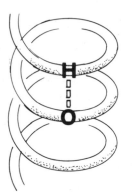 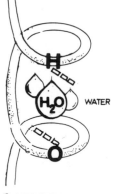 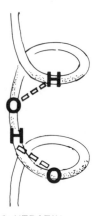

∝ KERATIN
Dry hair unstretched

β KERATIN
Wet hair stretched

β KERATIN
Stretched position

Heatsetting (dry setting)

Heatsetting, which is carried out on dry hair, works in a similar way. In this instance the hydrogen bonds are broken by the heat rather than water but the hair stretches to form beta keratin as before. The hair must be allowed to cool whilst still under tension so that new hydrogen bonds which will maintain the curl will be formed.

LOSS OF SET As soon as the 'set' hair becomes wet again or absorbs atmospheric moisture it changes back to the ∝ keratin condition and the set is lost. Because hair is hygroscopic (see page 73), the set will be affected by the level of humidity (the amount of water in the atmosphere). The greater the humidity the more water will be absorbed by the hair and therefore the quicker the set will be lost. The level of the humidity in the salon can be very high because of evaporation of water from sinks, hair, towels, etc. Good ventilation can control the level of humidity.

Hair setting aids such as setting lotions, hair gels, mousses and lacquers help to retain the set since they reduce the amount of water absorbed from the atmosphere by the hair.

METHODS

Shampooing

Make sure you select the appropriate shampoo and shampoo according to Chapter 6.

During the hair, scalp and skin analysis (see Chapter 5) you will have already decided whether or not the client needs a conditioner after shampooing. If she does need one, recommend it before taking her to the washbasin. Conditioners not only help damaged hair, but replace lost lubricant (the hair's natural grease — sebum). They are used after shampooing and after any excess water has been squeezed out of the hair.

Always check the manufacturer's instructions. Some conditioners have to be left on the hair, some rinsed out immediately, whilst others are left on for a few minutes and then any excess is rinsed out.

Combing the hair

Use a rake comb and disentangle the hair working from nape to forehead and points to roots (see page 87).

The hair may be combed at the washbasin after shampooing, or during the application of conditioners, but remember to check that the client is comfortable.

Setting and styling aids

During the hair analysis (see page 65), a decision will have been made as to whether a setting aid will be appropriate for the client's needs.

Special preparations are made to suit the correct styling technique.

Always read the manufacturer's instructions to check this. For example, setting lotions **should not** be used for blow drying as the hair becomes sticky and difficult to manage.

Always apply setting lotion and styling aids in a controlled manner. Setting lotions (especially those with added colour) are best applied to small sub-sections of the hair with a bowl and brush. To use mousse, first shake the can, then spray an amount the size of a small orange on to your palm, and apply evenly to the hair with your fingers.

Sectioning and winding the hair

After disentangling the hair and deciding the appropriate method of styling (see page 65), the hair must then be sectioned.

Sectioning allows you to work methodically and without being muddled.

The size and areas of sections will depend upon the equipment to be used — for example, pin curling needs small square sections, but natural drying will need much larger sections.

The sections must not be haphazard or untidy. Large sections should be secured with either section or butterfly clips.

Firstly, comb the hair into style using a setting comb then draw a clean line with the end of the comb along the scalp. The hair should then be parted. Hold the hair apart with one hand, then comb the hair down either side to create a clean parting.

Continue to part the hair in four directions for roller or pin curl sections, or in two directions for blow drying.

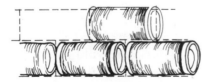

Sections for pin curls

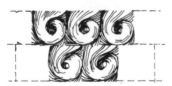

Sections for rollers

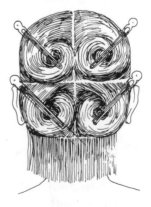

Sectioning for blowdrying

Setting (in pli)

Important factors to consider when setting in 'pli' are:

1 The hair must be clean.
2 The hair must be thoroughly wet.
3 Springy hair will take a tighter set than limp hair.
4 Rollers, pins and clips must be fastened securely, but remember metal equipment (straight pins and double pronged clips) will conduct heat and if they are touching the client's scalp or face, they will burn. If the set is too tight (too curly), then an incorrect choice of rollers was made, probably they were too small. Always ask the client how tight she would like the set to be.
5 The set must be thoroughly dry or it will fall or droop very quickly. All plis should be allowed to cool for 2-3 minutes before combing out.
6 If the hair is very long and thick then the set may also drop very quickly. Normal setting is done by the croquignole methods, i.e. wound from points to roots.

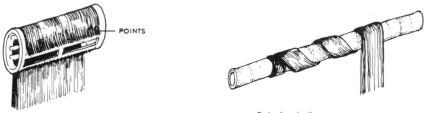

Croquinole winding   Spiral winding

Long hair may benefit from being set by spiral winding so that the curl at the root only turns around the roller once and produces tighter curl or wave movement near the roots.

7 Always make sure the ends are wound smoothly round the rollers during setting or they will become frizzy — these frizzy ends are called 'fish hooks'.

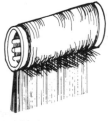

Overlapping ends   Result 'Fish Hooks'

8 In countries with damp atmospheres (especially the UK) cohesive sets tend to drop quickly because hair is hygroscopic and absorbs atmospheric moisture. This is a good reason for selling setting aids, e.g. mousse or setting lotion, to clients, both in the salon and for retail use.

To ensure a good result the following procedures must be used:

ROLLER SETTING Rollers are used to create volume in the finished dressing.
The roller size chosen for each pli will vary according to:

1 The style chosen.
2 The amount of curl already in the hair.
3 The length and amount of hair.
4 The elasticity in the hair, i.e. some hair has very little elasticity and needs smaller rollers than usual.

TECHNIQUES Generally rollers are positioned in the direction of the style intended. Look at the natural fall of the hair; a set will last longer if it is in the same direction.
Use a tail comb to take a sub-section of hair slightly smaller than the size of the roller.
It is easier to start at the top of the head, but always plan your pli in your mind before starting. Think about which size of rollers will be used on which area of the head and where the pin curls will be placed.
Once the section has been taken, comb the hair smoothly and evenly, without using any undue tension. Take the roller and wind the hair evenly and cleanly down to the scalp so that it sits on its base. Secure with a straight pin.

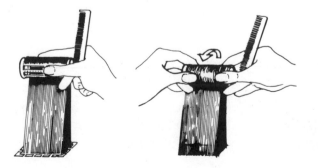

Inserting a roller

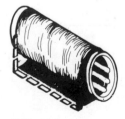

Roller on base

Remember not to allow the pins to touch the scalp or face.

Never place the rollers in straight rows or at right angles to the front hair line as this will cause breaks in the dressing, and is difficult to conceal whilst combing out.

PIN CURLS Pin curls are used to produce both curls and waves in a finished dressing. They are usually secured with double pronged clips, but care must be taken in securing them so that they are not distorted.

Square sections are usually taken with a tail comb and the hair must be combed smoothly with even tension.

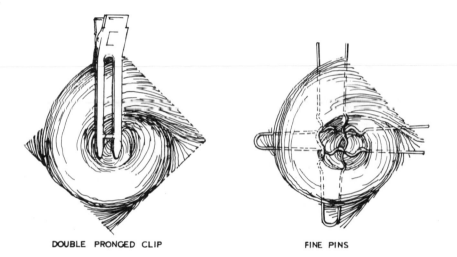

DOUBLE PRONGED CLIP   FINE PINS

Securing Pin Curls Depending on the direction of the intended finished curl — the hair must be combed in the opposite direction before curling.

Combing the hair from the roots is known as the root direction, the section of hair is then curled from the points (or ends).

Types of curl

STAND-UP BARREL CURL This curl is used for controlled volume instead of a roller. If complicated plis (see examples) are used, then sometimes a roller is too large for the section. A stand-up pin curl may be used.

Some plis are completed with stand-up pin curls.

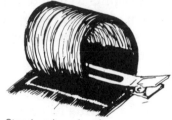

Stand up barrel curl

FLAT BARREL SPRING CURLS   These open pin curls produce soft movements.

If one row of pin curls is placed in one direction, and the next row is placed in the opposite direction, it is called **reverse pin curling.** These curls will brush out to create wave movement.

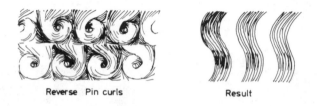

Reverse Pin curls   Result

CLOCKSPRING CURLS   These are flat pin curls with a closed centre. The points of the curl form a small closed circle with each loop of the curl becoming larger.

They are normally used in the nape area to produce tight curls.

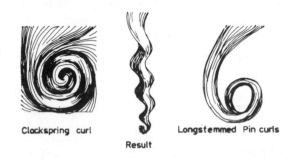

Clockspring curl   Longstemmed Pin curls

Result

LONG STEMMED PIN CURLS   These are useful for creating soft curl results around the hairline. As only the points are curled, they are often secured with special sticky tape to the skin.

Fingerwaving

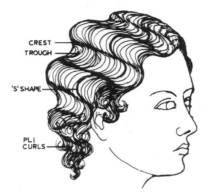

CREST
TROUGH

'S' SHAPE

PLI
CURLS

Fingerwaving is the moulding of hair to form wave movements. This is sometimes called water waving and employs a technique to produce a series of 'S' shaped movements in the hair. Setting aids help to hold the waves in place.

It is best to use unlayered hair, and to use the natural fall, or parting (see page 131).

The hair must be thoroughly wet for this technique, and the wide teeth of a setting comb are used with the index and middle fingers to hold each wave in place.

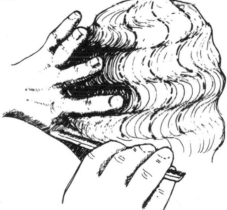

It is difficult to join the waves together, so it is better to work from the natural parting (or the front hairline) down, and to work along the head, thus completing one half of the 'S' shape before starting the next half of the 'S' shape.

The line formed between each curved trough is called the **crest** and the curve between each crest is called the **trough**.

As seen in diagram above, pli curls at the edges may complete the style.

The hair is then secured by a hair net and dried under a hood dryer. It may then be carefully brushed through to complete the dressing.

VARIATION PLIS   Italian boy

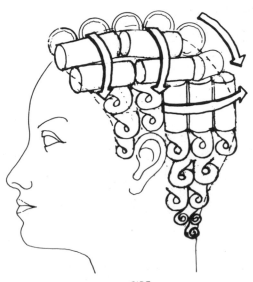

SIDE

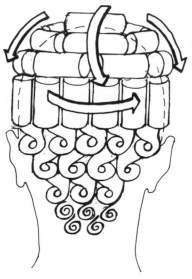

REAR

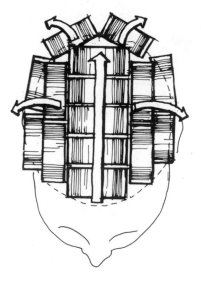

TOP

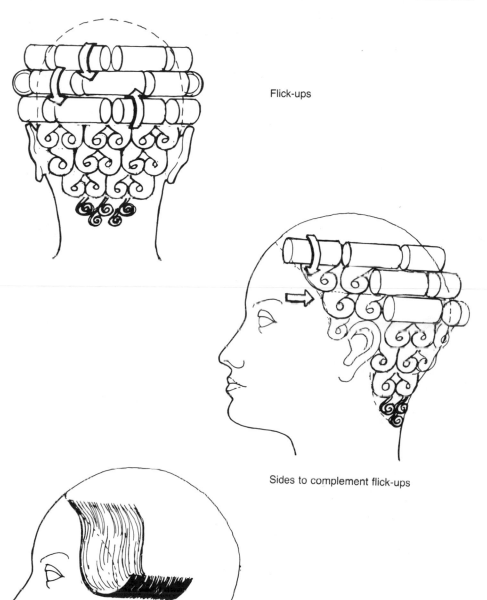

Flick-ups

Sides to complement flick-ups

Side flick-up

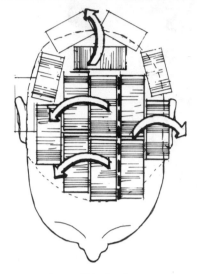

Long Side Parting

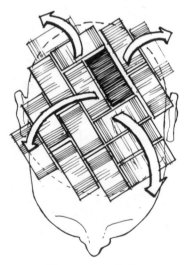

Forward on to Face

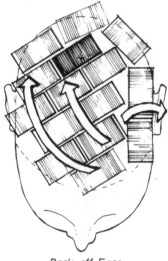

Back off Face

After completing any one of the pli's, secure the hairnet on the client's hair and secure some ear shields. Then, check that you have pre-heated the hood dryer.

Check that your client can use the dryer controls safely and make sure that she is comfortable. Clients are normally offered refreshments and magazines to read during this time. If the salon charges extra money for refreshments, be sure to mention this to the client beforehand.

BLOW DRYING/STYLING

A good, professional blow dry will last as long as hair that has been set in pli, but medium to thick textured hair with a slight inclination to wave is the best type of hair to blow dry. Well cut hair in good condition gives the best results.

Always check the cables, plug sockets and dryer connections for safety before use. Hand held dryers have an air intake grill at the back which must be regularly cleaned to remove dust and fluff, otherwise they will become dangerous and overheat.

Techniques

Rough dry the hair with a towel to save drying time (except for very curly, very fine or very short hair).

Place the hair in the direction of the finished style then section according to diameter of the brush chosen (flat, vent or circular). Very short hair need not be sectioned.

The root area is normally dried first and to increase volume direct over the mesh of hair, and direct the airflow to the roots.

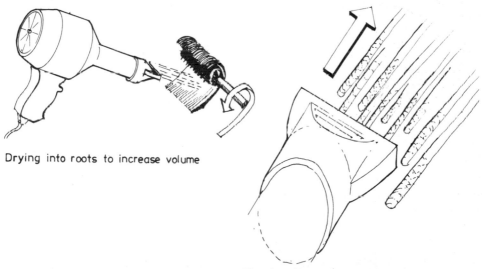

Drying into roots to increase volume

Keeping the cuticle scale flat

Keep the dryer moving to prevent burning the hair or the scalp. Make sure that each mesh of hair is thoroughly dry before taking the next section. Always lift the hair whilst removing the brush to prevent tangling.

You should work from roots to points keeping the cuticle scale flat. This will produce a shiny, sleek result.

Keep the airflow controlled to prevent disturbing the hair already dried. Hairdressers with long hair must keep it tied back. Remember cold air is drawn in through the back of the dryer — and long hair could get sucked in too!

The hairdryer is held in one hand and the brush in the other during blow waving, but the flex may not always stretch around the client — so learn to use both hands to hold the dryer at alternate times. Take care not to allow the flex to trail across the floor or over the front of the client — remember water and electricity together are dangerous!

Try to keep an even tension on the hair but do not overstretch the hair. If the dryer is held in one place for too long the hair may become over-dried and you could also burn the client's scalp.

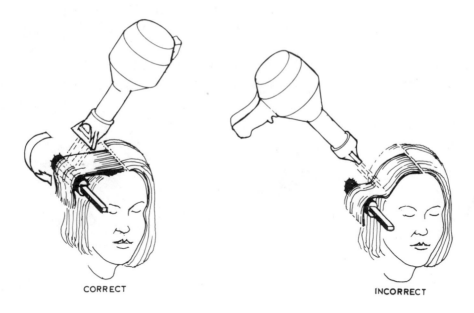

CORRECT   INCORRECT

Hairdrying brushes

FLAT BRUSHES These are good for smooth finishes, but difficult to use to achieve curled results.

VENT BRUSHES These are quick and easy to use, but can become tangled in the hair. They are good for breaking up the style to produce a soft effect.

CIRCULAR BRUSHES These are useful for producing a curled effect. The smaller the brush, the smaller the finished curl result.

Always allow each section of the hair to cool, then carefully remove the brush, before starting to dry the next section.

Blow waving

You should use a metal comb with wide spaced teeth for blow waving, and start at the front hairline.
    Use a nozzle attachment to concentrate the air flow of the hairdryer.
    The air flow from the hairdryer is directed along the wave crest in the direction of the movement.

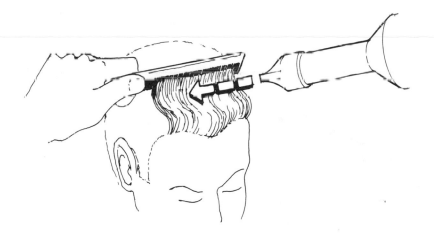

Natural drying

Certain hairstyles are better dried without too much disturbance, e.g. new perms. Equipment such as free standing or hand held infra-red dryers will dry the hair well. A special hand dryer attachment called a diffuser may also be used with care.

Scrunch drying

This is a method of blow styling using the hands and fingers instead of brushes. A diffuser attachment may be fitted to the hand dryer so that larger sections of hair can be dried than normal. The finished result is often very soft and casual, and the outline shape should be created by using an afro comb.

HEATED STYLING EQUIPMENT — for Heatsetting (dry setting)

Checking equipment

Always check cables, plug sockets and connections for safety before use. The appliances are cleaned with cotton wool and methylated spirit — **never** immersed in water! Heated styling aids are used on dry hair before finally dressing out. Many varied shapes and looks can be achieved for both everyday styles and for special occasions.

Electric tongs

ROD — STAND — GROOVE

Tongs or curling irons are used to produce a variety of effects from curls and waves to ringlets. Although they are thermostatically controlled, they can burn, so precautions are necessary. If used close to the client's scalp or skin, a heat resistant comb must be placed underneath for safety.

Some flexes have a swivel action to prevent twisting the cables, which can wear away and become dangerous.

Always use the stand to prevent work surfaces from becoming

scorched, and plastic surfaces, such as equipment trolleys, from being melted!

Light coloured hair can become discoloured and scorched if the heat is too strong from the tongs. Likewise, remember to allow the tongs to cool down before replacing them in cupboards or bags.

CURLING   To produce curls turning under, use the groove on top and the rod underneath. To curl hair up, use the groove underneath and the rod on top. Whilst curling long hair the tongs must be ventilated which means opening and closing the irons to prevent scorching the hair.

WAVING   Using tongs to produce waves is called **iron waving.** The finished effect is similar to finger waving (see page 109).

To blend waves together always take a small section of the previously waved hair whilst blending in.

RINGLETS   These are produced by taking small sections of hair and inserting the tongs near the root area. The hair is then wrapped smoothly around the tongs to produce a ringlet. The tongs must be removed carefully so as not to disturb the shape.

Hot brushes

Hot brushes are easier to use than tongs, but have a limited range of effects. Again, they are thermostatically controlled, and the flex may have a swivel action to prevent twisting.

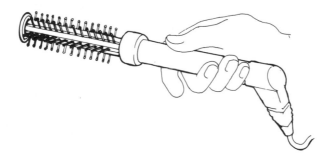

As with tongs, the ends must be wrapped clearly around the brush to prevent 'fish hooks'. Independent hot brushes are available which have no cable or flex, and are heated by butane gas or batteries.

Crimping irons

These are used on straight hair to produce a series of straight lines. They will create volume, making the hair appear thicker, and are useful for long hair.

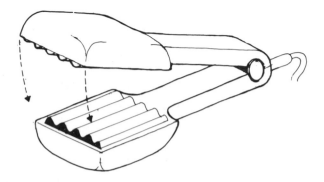

Heated rollers

These special rollers are heated by individual heating elements, and must be pre-heated for several minutes before use. The method is the same as for setting, using slightly larger sections, but the rollers must be allowed to cool down in the hair before being removed.

Each roller has its own special clip size which will only fit that roller. Some clients do not like heated rollers because they can tear the hair whilst being removed. However, special rollers are available which adhere to the hair without sharp spikes.

Sectioning

The amount of curl, length, density and thickness of the client's hair will determine the size of sections taken for various effects. Always think about the completed dressing before using any heated equipment, for example it may be better to pull long hair on to the top of the head and secure it, before curling it into ringlets.

Safety

Never over-stretch the hair, especially whilst dressing long hair, as too much strain can cause thinning, especially around the hairline. This is known as **traction alopecia** (see page 72). If the heated styling equipment is left in the hair for too long the hair may become over-dried and difficult to handle. Clients often complain of the effects of tongs, hot brushes and heated rollers during home use. If their hair is excessively dry, recommend that they have a soft body perm (see Chapter 10), or a series of conditioning treatments (see Chapter 9).

DRESSING (OR COMBING) OUT

Cooling the hair

After setting the hair in pli, blow drying or using heated styling equipment, the hair must be allowed to cool thoroughly before dressing out. The style will last much longer, especially if styling aids such as setting lotions, mousses or gels have been used.

Equipment

See pages 94-98 for the choice of equipment available for use during combing out.

Generally nylon and plastic tools tend to create more static electricity (causing flyaway hair) than do metal ones.

Open-tufted brushes are useful for the initial brushing of the hair but can separate the hair too much if a smooth finish is required.

Combs with fine teeth are useful for back-combing, and tail combs or straight pins may be used to lift the dressing to produce a uniform shape.

Section clips or double pronged clips help to flatten springy hair and hairspray may be applied to keep the shape. Remember to remove these clips immediately or the effect may be distorted.

Dressing aids

Always ask clients if they would like either dressing cream or hairspray before dressing out, and if there is any extra charge be sure to tell them.

DRESSING CREAMS Dressing creams are applied to dry hair before completing the dressing. They are made from mineral oils, and coat the outside of the cuticle scale to produce a shine on the hair, and are available as aerosols, creams or solids. (Beware — some hair colour restorers are similar to solid dressing aids.) Always use dressing creams sparingly as the hair may quickly become too greasy.

LACQUERS AND HAIRSPRAYS These used to be made from a shellac/acetone solution which was difficult to remove, both from the hair and from hairdressing equipment.

Nowadays, they are made from synthetic resins such as **Polyvinyl Pyrrolidone** (PVP) (this is also used in setting lotions).

Some hairsprays are coloured and used for special effects. Others are available with metallic particles (glitter) — but beware. If these are not removed before chemical treatments such as perms, tints or bleaches, then steam and breakage could occur.

Methods of dressing out

Some clients prefer a perfectly finished dressing, whilst others like a more casual result. Whichever the case it must be professional and suit the client's needs. The final dressing is what the client is paying for — so *make sure* that she is satisfied with the result.

If the hair has been set in pli or styled with heated styling aids, then it is necessary to brush the hair in all directions to remove roller marks.

After setting the hair should then be brushed in the direction of the pli, and back combed or back brushed, only if necessary.

BACK BRUSHING AND BACK COMBING This is a practiced technique and works because the cuticle scales are pushed apart and tangle with each other.

Tapered hair is easier to back comb or back brush than is club cut hair (see Chapter 8).

To remove back combing and back brushing always use an open-tufted brush or a comb with wide spaced teeth and start at the points of the hair, working towards the roots. Do not tear the hair.

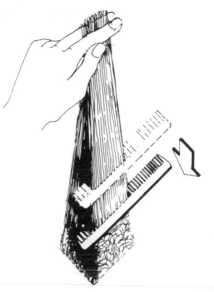

Backcombing technique

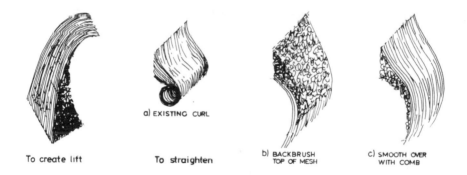

To create lift   To straighten

a) EXISTING CURL

b) BACKBRUSH TOP OF MESH

c) SMOOTH OVER WITH COMB

See Chapter 14 for descriptions of completed dressings to suit various face shapes.

Completion

Always stand a distance away from your client to check the finished result and shape. Look for any breaks in the dressing, and smooth over if necessary. Check the overall shape, looking at the back, sides and front. Does the front frame the face properly? If not, correct it (see Chapter 14).

Remember that the client only sees this area. **It is the most important part of the dressing.**

Hairspray and aerosol dressing creams may now be used to finish the work and to hold the shape. Use a lacquer shield to protect the client's face, and spray the hair from a distance of 30 cm for an even, controlled effect.

TEMPORARY HAIR STRAIGHTENING

Setting (wet)

Hair may be set, often with the use of setting aids (see Chapter 7), with large rollers to achieve a softer result.

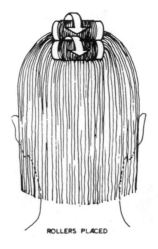

ROLLERS PLACED

The hair may be wrapped, where two rollers are placed on the crown area, and thus the remaining hair is combed smoothly around the head. The hair must be kept wet or styling aids applied, and kept in place with section clips.

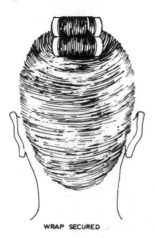

WRAP SECURED

You should use a hairnet and dry the hair under a hairdryer. Brush the hair through and finish with either tongs or a hot brush. Hair may be blow dried to achieve a smooth finish. Keep the hair wet and use styling aids (see page 100) and large shaped brushes to decrease the curl.

Setting (dry)

Hot brushes and electric tongs are useful for smoothing out and stretching over curly hair. Manufacturers also make special electric straightening irons for use on long hair.

Hot combs are often used for negroid hair but can be very damaging. They are heated and combed through the hair to produce a smooth effect.

MULTIPLE CHOICE QUESTIONS

1 Dressing mirrors are usually:
  - (a) concave mirrors
  - (b) convex mirrors
  - (c) plane mirrors
  - (d) refracting mirrors

2 Which of the following will destroy a cohesive set?
  - (a) a humid atmosphere
  - (b) sunlight
  - (c) a cold atmosphere
  - (d) a dry atmosphere

3 The term 'hygroscopic' means:
  - (a) quick drying
  - (b) absorbs moisture from the air
  - (c) tapering hair
  - (d) over stretched

4 When hair is stretched the following change occurs:
  - (a) β keratin becomes α keratin
  - (b) α keratin becomes β keratin
  - (c) the polypeptide chains break down
  - (d) β keratin becomes γ keratin

5 Setting lotions help to maintain a cohesive set by:
  - (a) reducing the amount of water taken up by the hair
  - (b) causing a film of water to coat the hair
  - (c) sticking the hair together
  - (d) unlinking the hydrogen bonds

6 Which of the following factors will increase the rate of evaporation?
  - (a) lower temperature
  - (b) high humidity
  - (c) still, unmoving air
  - (d) higher temperature

7 Many hair setting sprays contain the plastic:
  - (a) polyvinyl pyrrolidone
  - (b) protein hydrolysates
  - (c) pectin
  - (d) hexachlorophene

8 Open-tufted brushes are used to disrupt the pli because they:
  - (a) are only used on dry hair
  - (b) penetrate hair meshes more easily
  - (c) are made of natural fibre
  - (d) are easy to hold

9 When drying the pli, care must be taken to prevent scalp burns caused by:
   (a) hair pins touching the scalp
   (b) hair being sucked into the dryer
   (c) hair wound too tightly around curler
   (d) setting lotion touching the scalp
10 What is crocquinole winding?
   (a) winding from roots to points
   (b) reverse pin curling
   (c) hair in 'pli'
   (d) winding from points to roots
11 When rollers are placed at right angles to the front hairline, this produces:
   (a) lift at the roots
   (b) a smooth style
   (c) a side parting
   (d) breaks in the dressing
12 Reverse pin curls dress out:
   (a) in wave movements
   (b) in clock spring curls
   (c) in ringlets
   (d) in stand-up barrel curls
13 Hair is blow dried underneath the mesh:
   (a) to increase curl
   (b) to produce a shiny sleek result
   (c) to create volume
   (d) to prevent tangling
14 Waves are formed in blow waving by:
   (a) drying along the wave crest in the direction of the movement
   (b) using circular brushes
   (c) drying against the direction of the movement along the wave crest
   (d) scrunch drying
15 Thinning of the hair caused by over-stretching is known as:
   (a) diffuse alopecia
   (b) stretched alopecia
   (c) strained alopecia
   (d) traction alopecia.

8
CUTTING

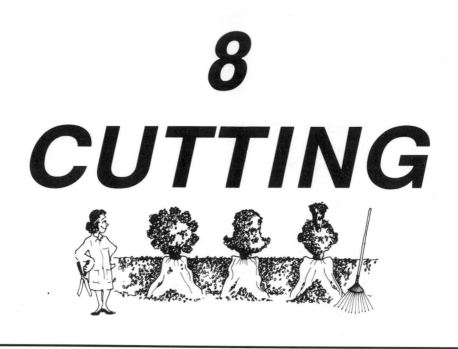

Cutting Analysis

More clients visit the hairdresser for cutting than any other service,
because it is impossible for anyone to cut their own hair as efficiently
as the professional hairdresser. A good haircut is the foundation of
every hairstyle and can change a client's view of themselves –
hopefully for the better!

The hairdresser can remove both length and thickness (bulk), and
create a completely new shape of style by cutting. It may be that the
client is quite happy with the same hairstyle as previously, and you
may need to gain their confidence before transforming them with a
new style.

A haircut must satisfy the client's requirements and a thorough
analysis is essential beforehand. The following cutting analysis chart
may be used as a guide and check list. It is important to do the
analysis before gowning up.

Cutting Analysis Check List

Name:

Address: Stylist's name:

Tel. no.   Date:

Factors to consider

1   client's requirements
2   face shape
3   body proportions
4   hair type
5   hair texture
6   abundance of hair
7   hair movement
8   natural growth patterns
9   hair quality and condition
10   scalp condition
11   client personality/dress/life-style
12   client limitations
13   suggested style
14   cutting techniques and reason
15   cutting method
16   styling considerations
17   finished result
18   home care advice

Preparation

Gowning up

There is nothing more irritating for a client than leaving a hairdressing salon covered in pieces of cut hair. Hairs not only fall down the back of clothing, but insert themselves into fabrics (especially sweaters) and are difficult to remove. Always keep a clothes brush (see page 47) at reception to remove hairs from the client's clothes after the gowns are taken off and before the bill is paid.

Normally close woven cotton or synthetic gowns are used to cover the client's clothes and shoulder capes are used around the client's shoulders. These must be kept clean by regular washing.

Towels may be used during wet cutting, but as cut hairs embed themselves in towels, it is more hygienic to towel dry the hair and use plastic shoulder capes to protect the client.

To prevent cut hairs from falling down behind the client's clothing insert either a strip of cotton wool or a neck tissue around the neck area. These are disposable, and should only be used once.

Wet cut hairs are especially difficult to remove from the skin, but the use of powder (often talcum) and a neck brush (or powder brush) makes removal of hair easier. These brushes must be regularly washed, dried and sterilized (see page 16).

Client requirements

Clients often select a photograph of a hairstyle beforehand (see Style Books, page 267) and wish to discuss the suitability of their hair for it. A compromise is usually possible when the following factors are taken into consideration.

FACE SHAPE   Clients are often aware of which style suits them and which styles do not, but they are not always certain of the reasons why. Personal face shapes can also change with time or weight gain or weight loss, so that different hairstyles may or may not suit someone at different times of their life (see Chapter 14).

BODY PROPORTIONS   This means not only the client's height and shape, but their proportions relative to a particular hairstyle. For instance, a long thin neck will be exaggerated by a short hairstyle, and

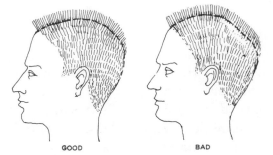

Head shape for 'Flat top'   GOOD   BAD

a large nose will be exaggerated by hair drawn back from the face. The shape of a person's head is very important, especially for very short haircuts where it is seen more clearly. The classic 'Flat top' hairstyle is often difficult to achieve because it does not match the client's head shape (see page 258).

HAIR TYPES Caucasian and Asian hair types are often cut according to their natural growth patterns. However, some Asian hair, notably Chinese hair, has very strong root growth. This hair will often appear much shorter than expected when cut, especially after wet cutting (see page 72).

Remember that hair will stretch up to one third of its length when wet (see page 102), so never cut off too much, or the dried hair will be shorter than both you and the client expected!

There are particular techniques used for either very curly Caucasian hair or Negroid curly hair. It is better to cut the hair dry, by shampooing first then natural drying (see page 115). An afro comb should then be used (see page 98) to disentangle the hair. Negroid hair often needs a moisturizing spray containing lubricant oils to help release some of the tangles.

The outline shape is very important when cutting Negroid hair. Clippers, scissor over comb or free-hand scissor cutting (with no combs) are highly skilled techniques. Scissors with long blades are easier to use, but whichever technique is chosen, the hair must continually be lifted out with the afro comb to create the shape.

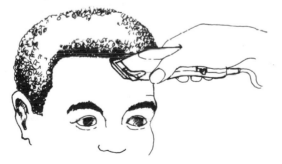

Electric clippers used to shape Negroid hair

OUTLINE SHAPING (e.g. 'Flat tops') Negroid hair is particularly good for outline shaping, but Caucasian and Asian hair may also be used.

Always check the natural hair growth pattern; it can work both for and against the haircut.

Negroid hair must first be blow dried into style, sometimes with the use of a styling aid (see page 100), then cut to shape. The completed shape must be checked against the background. This may be difficult to see if your clothes are patterned, so check the shape with either a back mirror or hold up a towel (of a contrasting colour) to see the outline shape. It is also useful to ask the client to slowly tilt the head from side-to-side while you check the shape.

HAIR TEXTURE This is the thickness or thinness of each individual hair. Some hair is so coarse and wiry that only extremely sharp tools (scissors and razors) used on fine sub-sections will cut it easily (see page 73).

ABUNDANCE OF HAIR Remember that it is possible for a head to have an abundance of fine or sparse but coarse hair. Generally fine hair will appear thicker when the ends are cut straight across (blunt or club cut) and coarse hair will appear thinner when it has been thinned with scissors or a razor and looks tapered.

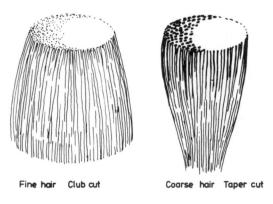

Fine hair   Club cut   Coarse hair   Taper cut

Tapered or thinned hair tends to curl or wave more because it has lost some of its weight (see page 92).

HAIR MOVEMENT Hair may be naturally curly or permanently waved to appear curly and the amount of curl or movement can be encouraged or discouraged according to the cutting technique, e.g.

club cutting and taper cutting. Generally hair that is all one length (see p. 142) will tend to curl less than layered hair because of its weight.

NATURAL GROWTH PATTERNS   The natural fall of hair is seen when it is in its alpha keratin state (see page 102), and best observed when it is wet. This is why most hairdressers prefer to cut wet hair.

Natural partings are found by combing the hair back from the front hairline and pushing gently with the palm of your hand. If you are cutting an all one length hairstyle such as a classic 'bob', then the natural parting is very important. The client must be able to manage the haircut herself at home and will find the natural parting in the same way as previously described. If it is in the wrong place, then the style will hang in an uneven way, with long ends straying down.

Other unusual hair growth patterns are a 'cow's lick' found at the front hairline, which makes straight fringes on fine hair difficult to cut, a 'double crown' which makes hair cut too short on the crown impossible to lay flat, and 'nape whorls' which make straight nape hairlines difficult to achieve.

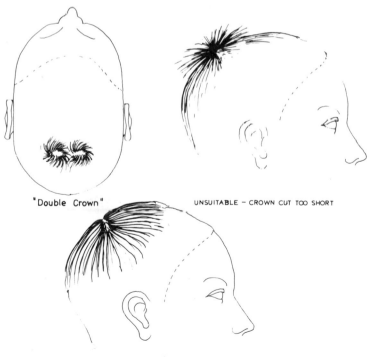

"Double Crown"   UNSUITABLE – CROWN CUT TOO SHORT

SUITABLE – LONGER CROWN HAIR

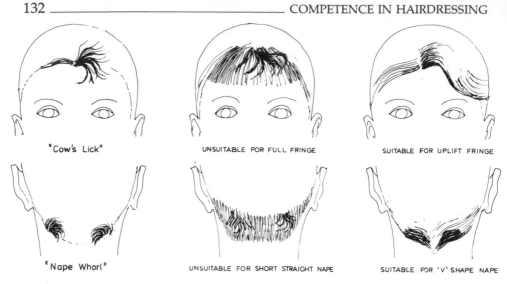

"Cow's Lick"   UNSUITABLE FOR FULL FRINGE   SUITABLE FOR UPLIFT FRINGE

"Nape Whorl"   UNSUITABLE FOR SHORT STRAIGHT NAPE   SUITABLE FOR 'V' SHAPE NAPE

HAIR QUALITY AND CONDITION   Although damaged hair can be made into better condition by conditioning treatments, very broken and split hair is better cut off.

Clients often find that they cannot grow their hair long. It may be because of their hair's life-cycle (see page 71) or simply that continued brushing, combing, tangling from windy conditions, tying back with elastic bands, back-brushing or chemical treatments such as perming, colouring and bleaching are causing their hair to tear, split and break off.

If the split ends (*Fragilatis crinium*) are only at the points of hair, then regular trimming (every 6 weeks) is necessary. However, if the hair is split and damaged along its lengths (*Trichorrexis nodosa*), then another cutting method is used. On dry hair take a small, square section of the damaged hair and twist it. Then rub the twisted strand of hair between your thumb and first finger so that the shorter, split ends stick out. These ends are easy to see as they are often white in colour. Hold the twisted hair firmly while you cut off the split ends.

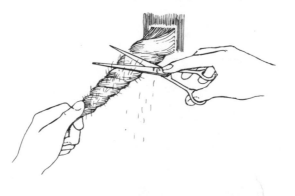

SCALP CONDITIONS Always check the scalp for cuts, abrasions, inflammation, infections and infestations (see page 66). Small abrasions are covered with collodion, but other non-infectious conditions such as Psoriasis and Sebaceous Cysts require special care when cutting.

Remember: cutting has no effect on hair growth, it just makes hair appear to be in a better condition.

CLIENT PERSONALITY, DRESS AND LIFE-STYLE The client's personality (extrovert or introvert), life-style (which will influence how much time they have to spend on their hair) and occupation are often reflected in her/his manner of dress (see page 93).

Never assume that because clients have chosen your salon for a haircut, that they wish to adopt your particular style. Some of the most *avante garde* salons which produce very high-fashion work, also have a large clientele who prefer simple, classic haircuts.

CLIENT LIMITATIONS Hair, scalp and body proportions and client personality and life-style limitations are all important factors to consider beforehand.

However, because cutting is one of the most regular sources of salon income – remember the client's time. Clients will tend to return to your salon if they are sure that they will have a good haircut, at a fair price, and within the time that they have to spare.

METHODS AND TECHNIQUES

Hair may be cut wet or dry. Some haircuts may take longer than others and the hair may begin to dry during wet cutting. A water spray (filled with warm water for the client's comfort) is then used to wet the hair (see page 100). Some techniques are best suited to wet hair and others to dry hair. For example:

Wet method   – razor cutting
Wet or dry method – club cutting
                      – taper cutting
                      – thinning
                      – point cutting
                      – clipper over comb cutting
                      – scissor over comb cutting

Tools

All cutting tools must be clean, sterile, sharp and in good condition.

SCISSORS Hairdressing scissors are expensive and finely engineered. They must never be used for anything other than cutting hair. All cutting blades must be kept dry and lightly oiled.

Sharp scissors, razors and clippers will cut hair cleanly, whereas blunt tools will tear the hair.

Scissors are available in various sizes from 100 mm to 180 mm in length from the tip of the blade to the handles. Many hairdressers prefer to use short scissors for precision cutting, but long scissors are useful for other techniques, such as cutting Negroid hair.

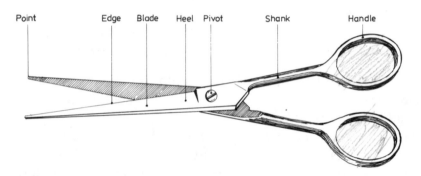

The pivot or screw holding the blades together is usually fixed tight by the manufacturer. If the scissors are accidentally dropped, not only the blades may be damaged but the pivot screw may become loose. The scissors must then be sent to a professional hairdressing scissor company to be mended or sharpened. As this is expensive always keep your scissors in their original protective case to prevent damage.

Hairdressers hold scissors with their thumb and third finger for maximum control whilst cutting.

To cut well, you must have good flexible wrists to be able to cut hair at every angle. Normally, whilst cutting, one blade is kept still, whilst the other blade is moved by your thumb. Practise opening and closing the scissors whilst rotating your wrist.

COMBS During cutting, the sub-section of hair to be cut is held in the fingers of one hand and the scissors in the other. To hold the comb at the same time the scissors are **palmed** for safety and the comb is held in the scissor hand.

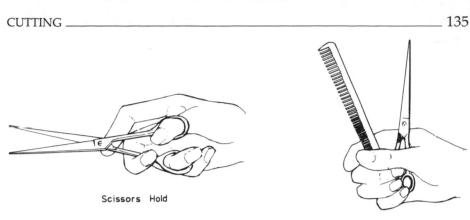

Scissors Hold

Palming Scissors

Salon (setting) combs and cutting combs (see page 48) are normally used during cutting, and a good flexible wrist movement is necessary again. During scissor over comb cutting, the fine, flexible cutting comb is used to continually comb and cut the hair in an up and down movement. To control the comb practise holding it both with the teeth pointed upwards and downwards.

Club cutting

This is the most common cutting technique used. However, it must be precise, and is often called **precision cutting**.

The sub-section of hair must be cleanly combed through and held with an even tension before cutting.

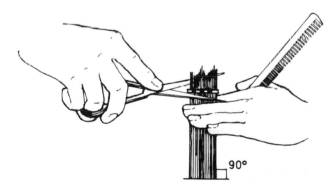

Hair may be club cut at any angle to the head according to the planned style.

Club or blunt cutting is normally done with scissors, but very occasionally an open razor is used. Clippers are also used to produce a club cut effect.

Taper cutting

Taper, slither or feather cutting will reduce both the length and bulk (thickness) of the hair. This technique is normally done on dry hair, and unlike club cutting (where the hair is cut over the fingers), the hair is cut underneath the fingers.

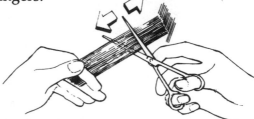

Tapering is a sliding, slithering backwards and forwards movement along a sub-section of hair.

Backcomb tapering is when the hair is backcombed first, then taper cut. The more backcombing the less tapering or thinning of the hair.

THINNING

Thinning is a cutting method which does not remove length, only bulk (thickness). Unlike tapering which is done with ordinary haircutting scissors, special scissors are used called **aesculaps**.

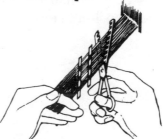

Thinning scissors with only one notched blade will remove less hair thickness than scissors with two notched blades. These scissors can remove quite a lot of hair, so it is best to use them on dry hair when the results can be seen easily.

A sub-section of hair is combed away from the head and the scissors are inserted underneath the fingers. To remove less bulk or thickness, backcomb the hair first.

Insert the scissors diagonally across the section and close them. Repeat this movement two or three times down the section until enough bulk has been removed.

Over-thinned hair can produce spiky ends which stick out, so never thin hair:

1 Around the hairline.
2 At the crown area.
3 Too close to the scalp.
4 Along any parting areas.

Many exciting and varied effects can be achieved with thinning scissors, and manufacturers have produced some new variations on the normal thinning scissors, with varying shapes of blades.

RAZORING

Razoring is generally done on wet hair because it is painful for the client if the hair is dry.

There are two types of razor which can be used; one is an open (sometimes called cut-throat) razor, and the other is a safety razor (sometimes called a shaper).

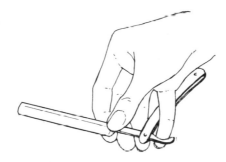

Open Razor Hold

OPEN RAZORS These must always be kept sharp, and in a barber's shop are sharpened on a special stone called a **hone**. This is called **setting** the razor.

The edge of the razor is then smoothed on a **strop** so that there are no rough edges. Hanging strops are made of leather and suspended from a wall, whilst solid strops are used on a work surface.

It is important to hold an open razor safely so that it does not close up on your hand whilst haircutting.

Open razors may be used to both shorten hair and to remove bulk, and are useful for hairline shaping. They must be kept sharp, dry and sterile and should be kept closed whenever they are not in use.

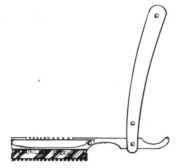

Safety Razor

SAFETY RAZORS   A hair shaper is similar to an open razor but uses a disposable blade, and therefore does not need either honing or stropping.

A safety razor will produce a feathered, uneven effect and is easier and safer to use than an open razor.

Keep safety razors dry and sterile and always covered with the guard. Replace worn disposable blades with sharp ones at frequent intervals.

Razors may be used either underneath or above the *wet* subsection of hair, and stroked towards the points in a scooping movement.

POINTING

Razors are useful for fashionable wispy, texturized looks, but these methods are easily achieved with scissors.

Pointing can be used to achieve feathered effects and to soften hard lines created by club cutting.

A sub-section of hair is taken and the scissors are inserted over the fingers to chip out small pieces at the ends.

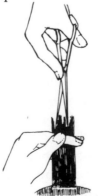

When larger pieces are chipped out of the ends of the hair it is called **texturizing**.

CHANNEL CUTTING

Channel cutting is used for high-fashion work, where small sub-sections of hair are cut very short and longer lengths are left in between. These longer pieces of hair can be gelled and coloured to stand up and create different effects. This works particularly well with Negroid hair.

SLIDE CUTTING

Slide cutting is particularly useful for joining short and long layers of hair. Very sharp scissors are needed and they are used under the fingers. On wet hair, one blade is pulled along the hair towards the points to create a long taper.

SCISSOR OVER COMB (shingling)

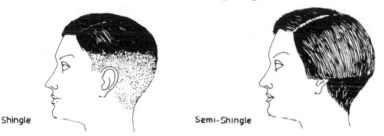

Shingle

Semi-Shingle

This very popular technique is highly skilled and mistakes can easily occur!

A cutting comb is used to pick up the hair and the scissors are kept parallel to the comb whilst cutting. The scissors and comb are moved up and out to form a graduation whilst cutting.

Clipper over comb

Clippers have two blades with sharp edged teeth. One blade remains fixed whilst the other moves across it. The distance between the blade points and the spacing between the blade points determine the closeness of the haircut. Some clippers have detachable heads with varying sizes of blades to produce different lengths of hair. These are numbered from 0000 (the closest) to 3 (the longest).

There are electric clippers which work from the mains and have a lead, and cordless clippers which are battery operated and rechargeable. Hand clippers are sometimes used where the handles are pulled together to move the cutting blade.

Always check that the clippers are safe to use, that the cutting teeth are not damaged and that the blades are both sharp and correctly adjusted.

Clippers are used to create a graduated effect in the same way as the scissor over comb method.

Hairline shaping

Some clients have difficult natural hair growths (see page 131) which can be overcome by hairline shaping. For instance, if the nape hairline grows into a 'V' shape and a square shape is required, then the neckhairs which grow in the opposite direction must be removed.

The hairline shape can be achieved by either using scissors, an open razor or clippers. This is sometimes called **lining out**.

Clippers are often used to create strong hairline shapes on men's hair – especially around the sideburn areas where the hair is coarser.

Scissors are used to create hairline shapes by resting the blades flat to the skin and opening and closing quickly. Normally the skin is stretched taut to prevent the scissors from cutting the skin, especially for mature clients with looser, wrinkled skin.

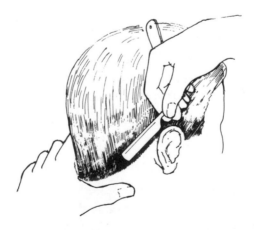

Hairline shaping

Hairline shaping is also used whilst cutting strong geometric shapes, to make the outline clean and precise.

Shampooing

For wet cutting, use the appropriate shampoo. You should shampoo the hair (see Chapter 6), condition if necessary and disentangle it.

PLANNED STYLES

There are three major style plans from which all other styles can be achieved.

1 The one-length cut.
2 The layer cut.
3 The graduation

After the initial haircutting analysis, all the important factors, including the client's face shape, head shape, natural hair growth and required style, will be in your mind. Remember to use this information during cutting as well as beforehand.

An open-tufted brush is often used during cutting to brush the hair in different directions to see how well the hair is falling into shape and to correct any imperfections. Always keep the water spray close at hand to redampen the hair if necessary.

Use the mirrors around the salon to check the shape of the client's haircut from various distances. Likewise, stand back occasionally from your client to see the effect.

Hand mirrors can also be used to check short graduations or bobs by placing directly underneath the hairline.

It is important not to pull the hair or use too much tension whilst cutting around the ears, as when the hair falls naturally it may be too short. Freehand cutting works better around this area.

Sometimes it is difficult to make both sides of a haircut even, so first make sure that your client is not sitting with legs crossed! Take small strands of hair from either side with your fingers from each hand and gradually slide your fingers to the ends. If the strands have been taken from exactly the same place at each side, then your thumbs should be level.

Remember to use the natural growths of the hair and work with the hair – not against it. The client has to manage the style at home without your professional help.

Sectioning

To work methodically through a haircut, it is better to create sections. These sections vary from style to style and the following diagrams are only a guide.

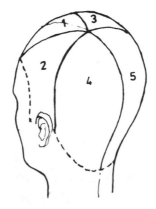

The sections may be secured with either section or butterfly clips (see page 96).

Keep the sub-sections of the hair narrow whilst cutting so that the cutting **guide line** can be clearly seen. Always comb the hair smoothly and hold the hair firmly whilst cutting or long ends will result.

Cutting guide lines

Guide lines may be taken either vertically or horizontally. It means that after the first guide line has been cut, then the next subsection to be cut should match it.

One length cut

This is where the hair is cut to fall at the same outside length. Hair often looks thicker when cut in this style. The front of this haircut can be varied by changing the angle of the guide line around the face (see page 252).

The back of this haircut can also be adapted to any length and for different shapes.

The guide lines are taken either horizontally or diagonally starting at the hairline.

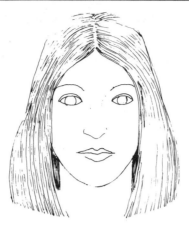

One length cut

Always cut a one length cut from the **natural fall** both from the parting and the crown area, combing the hair perfectly smooth and even.

To check that a one length cut is even ask the client to slowly move the head from side-to-side and back and forward. Any unevenness or long ends will be clearly seen.

Layer cut

A basic layer cut is where each sub-section of hair is of the same length. The weight and fullness of the style is evenly distributed, and it can be set, blow dried or dried naturally easily.

The outline shape of a layer cut is taken in the same way as for a one length cut. The guide lines may either be horizontal or diagonal. It is possible to achieve a layer cut by taking vertical guide lines and then cutting the outline shape (sometimes called the base line) afterwards.

The vertical guide lines for a layer cut are always taken at right angles to the head (90°).

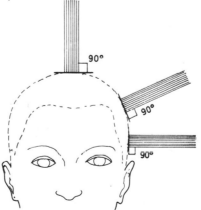

Vertical guide-lines

To check that the cut is even the layers are combed in the opposite direction to the way in which they have been cut. They must be perfectly even, with no long ends.

Graduation

A graduated haircut means that the layers vary in length from shorter to longer. It is also possible to have a one length cut and a graduation in the same haircut.

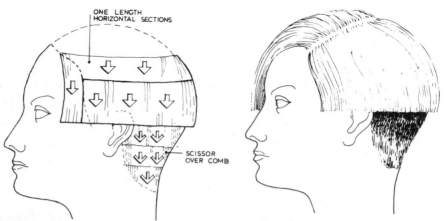

Longer layered hair is also a type of graduation, where the shorter layers are on the top of the head, and the longer layers are underneath.

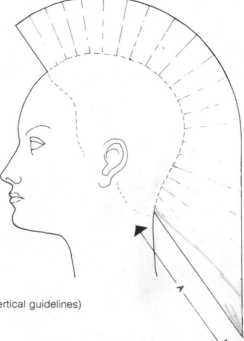

Long graduated haircut (vertical guidelines)

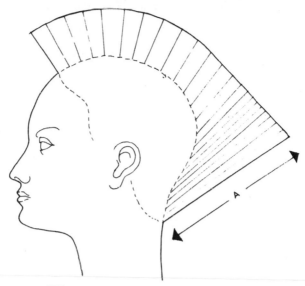

LONG LAYERS OVERDIRECTED

Sometimes it is difficult to blend or match long layers, so then the hair is **over-directed**, and pulled together.

Over-direction is a useful technique when cutting graduation in the layers. It can also be used for short cuts.

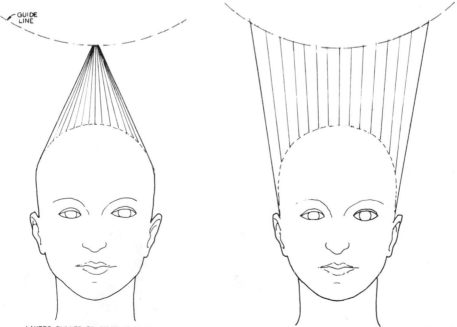

LAYERS PULLED TO FIRST GUIDE LINE   LAYERS COMBED UPWARDS TO FORM GRADUATION

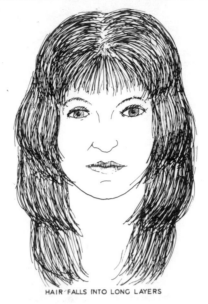

HAIR FALLS INTO LONG LAYERS

During layering, normally the first guide line is pulled across to match the next sub-section being cut. To over-direct the layers, all the sub-sections are pulled across to the first guide line.

The one length cut, layer cutting and graduation are all techniques which rely on the angle at which the hair is cut.

Combined with the other cutting methods and techniques such as tapering, clipper cutting, razoring, thinning, slide cutting, channel cutting and scissor over comb cutting – any haircut can be achieved.

Each haircut must be individually designed for the client using a combination of technical skill and design ability (see Chapter 14 and 15).

Undesirable effects following cutting

Cutting fault		Cause
Removal of too much hair	1	Incorrect analysis (page 126)
	2	Incorrect control of razor (page 137)
	3	Incorrect control of thinning scissors (page 136)
	4	Incorrect selection of cutting technique
Damage to hair (cuticle)	1	Blunt cutting tools (page 134)
	2	Infrequent use of water spray (page 141)

Cutting fault		Cause
Damage to skin or scalp	1	Incorrect scalp examination (page 133)
	2	Incorrect control of cutting tools (page 134) **NB** Always keep scissors directed away from ears and eyes. Always take special consideration towards children (see Chapter 14 and 15) and physically and mentally handicapped clients.
Imbalanced style	1	Incorrect choice of cutting tools and techniques (page 133-40)
	2	Ignoring natural growth patterns (page 131)
	3	Ignoring planned style (page 141)
	4	Unmethodical procedure (page 142)
	5	Incorrect cutting angles (page 142)
	6	Incorrect tension on the hair (page 135)
	7	Infrequent use of mirror (page 141)

SAFE PRACTICES

Removing hair cuttings

Hair cuttings should be removed with the neck brush from the client's face and neck areas during cutting. Any excess hairs clinging around the neck area should be removed as the cotton wool or neck strip is taken away, and extra hair brushed thoroughly off the skin.

Use the neck brush to remove any excess hair from the client's gown, so that when it is removed, hairs do not cling to the client's clothing.

Once the client is at the reception area, or if remaining at the dressing position for further service, then sweep up the hair. Loose hair cuttings can be hazardous and unhygienic, and must be swept up and placed in a covered container or burnt.

Accidentally cutting the client

If an accident does happen, keep calm, apologize to the client and using a sterile pad of cotton wool to apply pressure to the cut to stop the bleeding. **NB** Aids threat (see page 13). Small cuts may be covered with a sterile dressing, but larger cuts may need medical treatment.

Remember that the skin on the ear lobes is quite thin, and a small cut may bleed more than expected, so keep the pressure on it until the blood clots.

Accidentally cutting yourself

Many hairdressers cut themselves during haircutting (between the first and second fingers where the hair is held is the favourite place).

Stop whatever you are doing and excuse yourself from the client. Rinse the cut with water to remove any excess hairs or debris, then apply pressure with a sterile cotton wool pad until clotting occurs. Cover the cut with a sterile dressing, a material plaster works best, but make sure your skin is perfectly dry or it will not stick to your skin. Large cuts may need medical treatment, but it is better to dress the cut yourself because of the risk of infection.

MULTIPLE CHOICE QUESTIONS

1   A type of cutting which is used to reduce both length and bulk is:
    (a)   taper cutting
    (b)   thinning
    (c)   club cutting
    (d)   point cutting

2   Cutting makes fine hair appear:
    (a)   thinner
    (b)   more curly
    (c)   thicker
    (d)   tapered

3   If the hair is not combed smoothly during club cutting, then the hair may be:
    (a)   uneven
    (b)   asymetrical
    (c)   feathered
    (d)   symetrical

4   A cutting comb is used for:
    (a)   cutting short hair in the nape area
    (b)   thinning the hair
    (c)   tapering the hair
    (d)   point cutting

5   What effect does cutting have on hair growth?
    (a)   it makes the hair thicker
    (b)   it makes the hair grow more quickly
    (c)   it makes the hair more abundant
    (d)   no effect

6   What areas of the hair must **not** be thinned with Aesculaps?
    (a)   behind the ears
    (b)   under the crown
    (c)   above the ears
    (d)   hairline or parting areas

7   What piece of equipment is used to keep open razors sharp?
    (a)   a strop
    (b)   none – they are disposable
    (c)   a hone
    (d)   a set

8   For haircutting, scissors are normally held with the:
   (a)   thumb and third finger
   (b)   thumb and second finger
   (c)   thumb and first finger
   (d)   thumb and fourth finger

9   The size of clippers which gives the shortest haircut is:
   (a)   00
   (b)   001
   (c)   01
   (d)   0000

10   Another name for a shingle is a:
   (a)   flat top
   (b)   graduation
   (c)   an over-direction
   (d)   clipper over comb

9

TREATMENT CONDITIONING

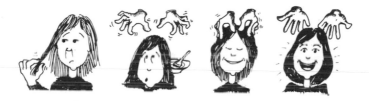

Many clients complain and say 'I can't do a thing with my hair at the moment!'

There are many reasons why this may be the case. It may be because of internal factors such as poor health, diet, hormonal changes, drugs, over or under activity of the sebaceous glands or perhaps stress.

Sometimes bad brushing and combing and overdrying the hair (**mechanical damage**) (see Chapter 7), or excessive perming, bleaching and tinting (**chemical damage**), or even **weather conditions** (sun, sea or wind) can be the cause. Many people shampoo their hair very frequently and this combined with regular chemical treatments, such as perms, hair-colours and highlights can make both the hair and the scalp become too dry.

You, the hairdresser, can help to restore the hair and scalp to a healthier state by offering the client a series of conditioning treatments, which combined with special scalp massages, will also help to relax the client.

GOOD AND BAD HAIR CONDITION

	Good Condition	Bad Condition
Surface condition	Cuticle scales lie flat and close together. Surface is smooth and shiny.	Cuticle scales are raised, open and may even be destroyed. Surface is rough and dull.
	A thin coating of sebum produces lustre and makes the hair more supple and less brittle.	The hair is more porous, so sebum is absorbed leaving insufficient on the hair to create lustre. Lack of sebum also reduces moisture content of hair and the hair becomes 'dry'. Hair chemicals are absorbed more easily which can result in internal damage.
Internal condition	The Chemical linkages in keratin are intact, and the hair is, therefore, strong and elastic and contains natural moisture	Some of the chemical linkages in keratin have been broken by strong chemicals, e.g. perm lotion, hydrogen peroxide. The hair loses moisture, strength and elasticity, i.e. becomes straw-like. Increased porosity causes the hair to swell and hold more water when wet, making it more difficult to dry.
Summary	Closed cuticle Shiny Lustre Non-porous Moisture content good Protein content good – Hair is strong and elastic	Open cuticle Dull Lack of lustre Porous Low moisture content – dry Low protein content – loss of strength and elasticity

ACIDITY AND ALKALINITY – THE pH SCALE

The degree of acidity or alkalinity of a substance is measured on the pH scale, which runs from pHO to pH14. pH7 is neutral (neither acid nor alkaline). pH values greater than 7 indicate alkaline substances, the greater the number the more alkaline the substance. pH values less than 7 indicate acid substances, the smaller the number the greater the acidity.

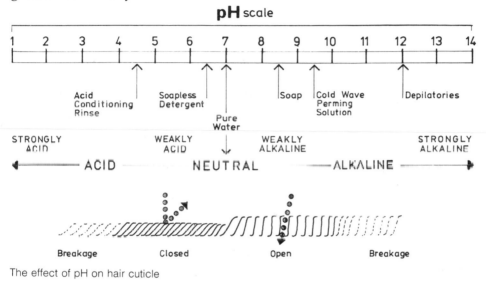

The effect of pH on hair cuticle

The effect of pH on the hair

Solutions that are slightly acid (pH4-7) will close the cuticle scales. This makes the outside of the hair smooth so that it reflects the light and looks shiny and healthy. Solutions that are slightly alkaline (pH7-10) will open the cuticle scales and make the hair swell. This will allow chemicals to enter into the hair cortex (e.g. perm lotion, tints, etc.) but makes the hair surface rough so that it scatters the light and looks dull and in poor condition.

Strong acids (pH0-4) and strong alkalis (pH10-14) will permanently damage the hair keratin.

pH balanced products

These have the same pH as the hair and skin (approximately pH5-6). They are useful after alkaline hairdressing treatments such as perming, tinting and bleaching to bring the hair back to its normal acid balance.

PREPARATION FOR CONDITIONING TREATMENT

Gowning up

Gown up the client with the appropriate gown, shoulder cape and towels, but remember that paper tissues may be needed around the client's neck to absorb any excess oils.

Discussion

It is possible that the client may have problems with both his/her hair (e.g. overprocessed, dry ends) and his/her scalp (e.g. naturally greasy hair roots and scalp condition) at the same time. If this is the case, deal with the worst problem first, then when it has been corrected, start to treat the second problem.

Complete client records are essential – here is an example of one.

		TREATMENT RECORD CARD			**Index No.**			
Name								
Address								
						Tel. No.		
Date	Hair condition	Scalp condition	Product used	Equipment used	Time	Other details	Stylist	

EXAMINATION OF THE HAIR AND SCALP

For a more detailed analysis, this chart may be a useful guide.

Treatment Analysis Check List

Name:

Address: Date:

Tel. no.

Reference to Record Card Index no.

Hair and scalp analysis

| 1 | Hair texture | Porosity | Tensile strength |

1 Hair texture   Porosity   Tensile strength

2 Previous chemical treatment

3 Shampooing frequency

4 Scalp disorders   Scalp condition

5 General health and diet/medication

6 Atmospheric exposure

7 Mechanical damage

8 Treatment aims

9 Products used

10 Method (e.g. massage, etc.)

11 Processing equipment

12 Development time

13 Result

14 Homecare advice

15 Special notes

16 Final effect after six treatments

A practical examination of the hair and scalp is always necessary as well as the previous discussion with the client. Any client with an infectious scalp condition should be tactfully referred to a doctor, and no hairdressing services should be carried out.

Some non-infectious conditions may be treated in the salon.

The differences between infectious and non-infectious scalp conditions are explained in Chapter 2, pages 11–14. (Details of non-infectious scalp and hair conditions may be found in Chapter 5, page 68.) Overleaf is a brief summary.

NON-INFECTIOUS SCALP AND HAIR CONDITION

	Name	Description	Cause	Treatment
S	Dandruff (Pityriasis Simplex)	Small, itchy, dry scales, white or grey coloured.	Overactive production and shedding of skin.	Oil conditioners conditioning creams, selenium sulphide or zinc pyrithione.
	Greasy dandruff	Dandruff and sebum which bind the scales together.	As above and overactive sebaceous glands.	Selenium sulphide or zinc pyrithione.
C	Greasiness (Seborrhoea)	Excessive oil on the scalp and skin.	Overactive sebaceous glands.	Spirits (alcohol).
A	Dermatitis	Red, inflamed cracks in the skin, often itchy.	Scale irritation may be caused by chemicals, e.g. perm lotions, detergents, paradyes, or by scratching.	Medical treatment.
L	Psoriasis	Thick, raised, dry silvery scales often found behind the ears.	Possibly hereditary, recurring in times of stress.	Medical treatment.
P	Alopecia	Baldness.	Many different causes.	Medical treatment.
	Sebaceous cysts	Large bumps on or under the scalp.	Retention of sebum from the sebaceous glands.	Medical treatment.

	Name	Description	Cause	Treatment
H	Split ends (*Fragilitas crinium*)	Split, dry roughened hair ends.	Harsh mechanical or chemical damage	Cutting, oil conditioners and conditioning creams.
	Hair breakage (*Trichorrhexis Nodosa*)	Hair roughened and swollen along the hair shaft.	Harsh chemicals (especially during perm winding if the rubbers are fastened too tightly). Mechanical damage (e.g. from elastic bands).	Test before treatment to see the extent of the damage.
A				
I	Distinct areas of white hair (canitics)	Lack of hair colour pigment – may be seen in young and older people.	Unknown.	Apply a permanent hair colour to match the natural hair.
R	Excessive hair growth (Hyper-trichosis or hirsuties)	Excessive hair growth in areas not usually covered, e.g. female faces – making some chemical processes, e.g. depilatory creams, dangerous if used near the eyes.	hormonal imbalances.	Electrolysis.

Analysis testing

Although most of these hair and scalp disorders are obvious visually, in the case of hair breakage due to harsh chemicals and mechanical damage, the **tensile strength** must be tested. This may be done by firmly holding the roots of a few hairs in one hand and the points in the other hand, and gently pulling the hair. This is also usually done during highlighting (see Chapter 12) to ensure that the hair is not being over-processed.

However, a manufacturer's **tensile strength meter** is more accurate as it tests the amount of elasticity in one hair. Hair normally stretches up to one third again of its original length and any more than that means that it has been over-processed.

If the hair has not been too badly over-processed, the normal oil or conditioning treatments are useful. However, badly damaged hair may need a restructurant.

TYPES OF CONDITIONER

Acid rinses

Weak acids, (pH4-5) such as ascorbic, citric and acetic acids are beneficial to the hair because they neutralize excess alkaline left over from hair treatments such as perming, bleaching and tinting, and thus restore the hair to its natural acid balance. The acids also close the cuticle scales which produces a smooth and shiny hair surface.

Oil conditioners

Vegetable oils, e.g. olive oil, almond oil, are used in hot oil treatments. The oil coats the hair and helps to prevent mechanical damage and loss of moisture. Hair is thus made soft, supple and shiny.

Conditioning creams

Conditioners are emulsions (see page 52) which contain ingredients (usually synthetic) which work in a similar way to sebum (the natural hair conditioner produced by the sebaceous gland). The exact formulation of the conditioner will vary according to the precise requirements but they are all designed to make the hair more manageable, elastic and glossy and some may help to preserve the set.

Deep-acting conditioners

Some conditioning creams are also **cationic** (having a positive electrical charge) which makes them stick to the hair shaft and remain there even after rinsing and drying. They are said to be **substantive**. They often contain **cetrimide** (a quaternary ammonium compound) which also has certain antiseptic properties and is an anti-static agent.

Restructurants

Restructurants contain **protein hydrolysates** (break down products of proteins such as keratin). If the hair is damaged some of these may enter the hair shaft, but usually they stick to the hair surface because of electrical charges (i.e. they are also substantive). They can be used as 'fillers', before perming or bleaching, to prevent loss of protein material during processing or as conditioners in after-perm and after-bleach conditioners. The surface of the hair is made smoother and more shiny but increase in strength is doubtful.

EQUIPMENT

Accelerator

(See page 44.) The heat from the infra-red light helps the hair to absorb conditioners and allows deeper penetration into the hair shaft. Do not leave the client under the accelerator for more than 15 minutes as you could burn the scalp (if the hair is not covered with a plastic cap).

Scalp steamer

(See page 44.) Steamers are extremely beneficial to use in conjunction with conditioning treatments as they help to swell the hair and raise the cuticle scales, thus allowing deeper penetration of the product into both the hair and scalp.

The steamer produces moist heat in the form of moist moving air through the evaporation of distilled water. Always check that the water reservoir is full before switching the steamer on, so that the heating element does not become over heated. Always check for safe wiring and connections before each treatment, and clean out thoroughly after use.

Switch the steamer on high a few minutes before you need to use it, then turn it down to the correct temperature whilst in use.

Applicators

Conditioning treatments may be applied directly from bottles filled with small nozzles, or by the use of bowls and sponges or brushes. If vegetable oils are used, they are best applied with a spatula with one end wrapped in cotton wool. The cotton wool can then be thrown away after use, this is because any excess oil left in sponges or brushes will affect other chemicals and may render them useless.

Always make sure you clean applicators thoroughly after use, and dry them properly.

Bowls

Similar size bowls as are used for applying permanent wave lotions, tints and bleaches are used for conditioning treatments. Always clean and dry them thoroughly.

Measures

Professional hairdressing measures are needed for accurately dispensing correct amounts of a product (see page 53). These too, must be thoroughly rinsed, cleaned and dried after use.

MATERIALS

Always follow closely the manufacturer's instructions during conditioning treatments, as the same product may be applied in a different manner for varying hair and scalp problems.

Acid rinses

After shampooing the hair and towel drying it, a citric or acetic acid rinse may be applied. Normally one third teaspoon of either acid is diluted into a pint of warm water, and rinsed through the hair using a jug. The hair need not be rinsed again with any more water, just towel dried.

Conditioning creams (external)

These may be applied with a bowl and brush to towel dried hair after shampooing.

Oils

Vegetable oils are applied to dry hair before it is shampooed. Oil is often warmed by placing a jug of warm water underneath the container which is holding the oil, making it easier to apply.

Spirits

These are used for greasy hair and scalp conditions (as in dry shampoos, page 82) and are specially prepared by various manufacturers. They help to suppress production of excess grease.

Specialist preparations

Many manufacturers produce complete ranges of shampoos, conditioners and home care treatments. It is very important to advise the client on the use of the product at home, as the treatments must be regularly used for a specific time in order to be effective. Your selling skills here are very important (see page 37).

Always follow the manufacturer's instructions and try to attend any specialist courses that are available. Some manufacturers give diplomas of competency in use of their products, which is useful for advertising the salon.

Some salons have their own brands of treatment ranges – complete with their own logo or motif (see page 283).

Restructurants

These are usually available in individual containers and are applied to towel dried hair. Apply them to the most damaged parts of the hair first and then to the rest of the hair. They are not usually rinsed out.

Cotton wool

Always use good quality cotton wool to apply products, and protect the client with dampened cotton wool strips around the hairline if the product is particularly runny.

Protective clothing

The client is gowned up to protect her/his clothes, and the hairdresser must also wear a suitable protective apron. If you need to wear professional hairdressing gloves whilst applying the conditioner, be sure to remove them before massaging the client's scalp – otherwise this can be very uncomfortable for her/him.

METHODS OF HAIR CONDITIONING TREATMENT

Shampooing

Most conditioning treatments are applied after shampooing with the manufacturer's recommended product. However, oils are always applied to dry hair.

Sectioning

Always disentangle the hair in the proper manner (see page 87) and take suitable size sections to work methodically. The size of the sub-sections will vary according to the product used and the length, texture and problem areas of the hair.

Application

Apply the product with either an applicator bottle (if specified by the manufacturer) or a bowl and sponge, brush or spatula and cotton wool, depending on which product has been selected. Use a rake comb to comb the product through the hair to distribute it evenly throughout the lengths.

Processing

Check the manufacturer's instructions for the correct processing time and method. Although steamers and accelerators are often used, some treatments are processed with a plastic cap covering the hair (to retain body heat) which may even be placed under a hood dryer.

Removal

Again, check the manufacturer's instructions for removing the product. Remember that some are not removed at all, whilst others may need one or two shampoos.

Removal of oil treatments

To remove oils always apply the shampoo before the water to form an emulsion and then rinse thoroughly from the hair before shampooing in the normal way.

Proceed with setting method

Continue by either setting, blow drying, natural drying or scrunch drying the hair.

Remember not to overdry the hair and undo your hard work!

METHODS FOR SCALP CONDITIONING TREATMENTS

Disentangling

Disentangle the hair properly (see page 83).

Application

Apply the product thoroughly to every part of the scalp area using either an applicator bottle, bowl and brush, sponge or spatula and cotton wool.

Scalp massage

This may be done by hand or by use of a vibratory machine.

CONTRA-INDICATIONS   Never massage the scalp:

1   When there are any infections or infestations present.
2   If there are any cuts or abrasions on the scalp.
3   If the scalp is inflammed or sore to touch.
4   If the client has any medical problems, even a high temperature, as with colds or 'flu.

HAND (MANUAL) MASSAGE   This is a relaxing treatment and should be done slowly in a calm atmosphere to relax the client. During the process the scalp becomes redder in colour (this is called hyperaemia) and the blood supply is increased to the hair follicle, which encourages hair growth.

MASSAGE MOVEMENTS
All massage movements should work from the top of the head down towards the nape to bring the blood supply back down towards the heart and to increase lymph drainage.

Effleurage   This is a stroking movement which begins and ends the massage procedure.

With your fingers spread slightly apart, and starting at the front hairline apply an even pressure and slowly slide your fingers through the hair down to the nape in one continuous movement. You should cover most parts of the scalp with your fingers, so that when you repeat the movement several times the client starts to relax.

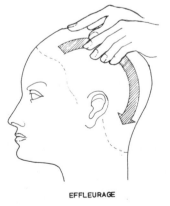

EFFLEURAGE

Petrissage   This is a deeper, kneading movement, using the pads of the fingers. It is sometimes called a rotary movement because it is similar to the one used for shampooing. However, whilst the fingerpads are still moved in a circular direction, the scalp should be picked up and kneaded.

People with a lot of thick hair often have a 'mobile' scalp which is easy to knead, but others with fine, thin hair may have a tight scalp which is more difficult to work with. Always ask the client if your massage is comfortable.

If you are unsure about the amount of pressure to use, try out the massage on your own scalp first to feel it.

During petrissage, start at the front hairline, knead around the top of the head and then gradually work towards the nape area. This massage may last for about 5 10 minutes.

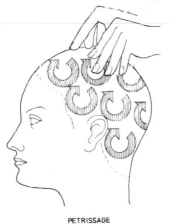

PETRISSAGE

Friction   This is a light, rubbing movement using the fingerpads. It is stimulating rather than relaxing and is not always carried out. It was the movement originally used during men's hairstyling whilst friction lotions (stimulating tonic lotions) were applied to the hair. It is only done for a few minutes, again working from front to back.

Vibro machines   This is an electrically operated vibratory machine which is used with its spiked applicator on the scalp.

It may be used after a hand massage for more scalp stimulation. After checking the plugs and cables, switch the machine on and it will begin to vibrate. Try the spiked applicator on the back of your hand to feel the amount of pressure.

Some clients enjoy the feeling, whilst others may find it irritating, so ask the client if it feels comfortable whilst having it used.

Start at the top of the head and gradually work down towards the nape area. Use small circular movements, lifting the machine out of the hair, whilst moving from one area to the next, so that the hair does not become tangled. You should only spend 5–10 minutes using this machine.

Upon completion, switch the machine off, remove the rubber spiked applicator, wash it thoroughly to remove any excess product, and then sterilize it. Carefully store the machine away.

Complete the massage with effleurage for a few minutes.

N.B. Never give scalp massage to clients with greasy hair and scalp conditions as you will over stimulate the sebaceous glands and make the problem worse.

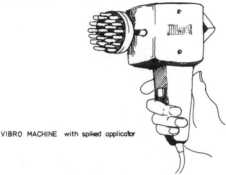

VIBRO MACHINE with spiked applicator

UNDESIRABLE EFFECTS FOLLOWING CONDITIONING TREATMENT

Faults	Cause and recitification
Tangled hair	1 Incorrect analysis of hair and scalp condition – reanalyze. 2 Incorrect choice of conditioner – re-analyze. 3 Incorrect removal of conditioner – rinse again.
Residue of conditioner left on hair and scalp	1 Incorrect removal of conditioner, rinse again.
Scalp damage	1 Incorrect analysis of scalp condition, re-analyze the scalp. 2 Incorrect use of vibratory machine. Try out the applicators on the back of your hand to test the pressure 3 Finger nails too long during hand massage. Cut them shorter.

MULTIPLE CHOICE QUESTIONS

1 Vegetable oil conditioners are applied:
   (a)   after the shampoo but before the final rinse
   (b)   after the final rinse
   (c)   as a dressing cream
   (d)   before the shampoo

2 The pH of an acid rinse is approximately:
   (a)   4–5
   (b)   7–8
   (c)   1–2
   (d)   9–10

3 Steamers are a useful aid to conditioning treatments since they:
   (a)   contain acids and so close the cuticle scales of the hair
   (b)   open the cuticle scales of the hair and allow deeper penetration of the conditioner
   (c)   dilute the conditioner
   (d)   repair damage to the polypeptide chains

4 A conditioner which is 'substantive':
   (a)   sticks to the hair surface because of electrical charges
   (b)   is anionic
   (c)   increases static electricity
   (d)   repels the hair because of electrical charges

5 The elasticity of hair damaged by perming or bleaching is:
   (a)   greater than normal hair
   (b)   less than normal hair
   (c)   the same as normal hair
   (d)   reduced during conditioning treatments

6 The 'tensile strength' of hair can be measured by:
   (a)   pulling the hair out
   (b)   a volt meter
   (c)   pulling the hair between the fingers
   (d)   a strand test

7 Bleached hair which appears dull would benefit from:
   (a)   a cold rinse
   (b)   a warm rinse
   (c)   an alkaline rinse
   (d)   an acid rinse

8   After a hot oil treatment:
     (a)   the shampoo should be applied before wetting the hair
     (b)   no shampoo should be used
     (c)   the hair should be shampooed in the normal way
     (d)   a shampoo containing oil should be used

9   The natural hair conditioner produced by the body is:
     (a)   sweat
     (b)   sebum
     (c)   cetrimide
     (d)   serum

10   The effect of an acid rinse on the hair is to:
     (a)   repair the polypeptide chains
     (b)   remove the cuticle scales
     (c)   open the cuticle scales
     (d)   close the cuticle scales

11   Split ends (*Fragilitas crinium*) are best removed by:
     (a)   a restructurant
     (b)   hot oil
     (c)   cutting off
     (d)   conditioning creams

12   Restructurants contain:
     (a)   hydrolysed protein
     (b)   hydrolysed polysaturates
     (c)   hexachlorophene
     (d)   ascorbic acid

13   Dressing creams contain:
     (a)   polyvinyl pyrollidone
     (b)   a mineral oil
     (c)   acetic acid
     (d)   sebum

14   Petrissage is a:
     (a)   soft circular movement
     (b)   sharp frictional movement
     (c)   soft stroking movement
     (d)   deep kneading movement

10

PERMANENT WAVING AND STRAIGHTENING

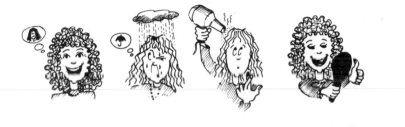

Permanent waving and curling is a technique used to **permanently** change the shape of the hair. When the hair continues to grow, its natural shape is seen at the roots or re-growth area.

Cold permanent waving is when permanent waves are lotioned, processed (sometimes with extra heat) and oxidized. Ordinary cold perms, acid perms and tepid perms are in common use today. There are many different techniques and winding variations to suit specialist equipment to achieve modern, varied effects.

Hot permanent waving was invented at the beginning of the 19th Century and this sometimes took ten hours to complete! Special lotions were applied and heat was used to process them, but no oxidizer was needed.

THE EFFECT OF PERMANENT WAVING ON THE HAIR

Perming involves changes in the chemical structure of keratin, the hair protein. This is why it has a permanent effect. It is the **di-sulphide linkages** in keratin (see page 70) which are affected by all the perming processes (cold permanent waving, heat perming and permanent straightening of hair).

Cold permanent waving

This is a two-stage process.

In the **first stage** (where perm lotion is used) some of the di-sulphide links which join the polypeptide chains of keratin together are broken. This is a **reduction reaction** (this means hydrogen is added) and is brought about by **ammonium thioglycollate** the reducing agent in the perm lotion.

The breakage of the linkages enables the hair to take the shape of the curlers or rods.

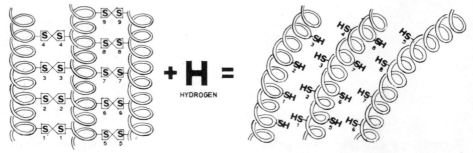

Breaking the di-sulphide bonds

Perm lotion also contains an alkali, **ammonium hydroxide**, which produces a solution of approximately pH9·5. The effect of this alkali is to open the cuticle scales of the hair and increase its porosity, thus allowing the perm lotion to penetrate into the cortex. However, this strong alkali has a damaging effect on the hair, and the hair is very delicate at this stage. Because of this, many of the modern perm lotions are only slightly alkaline or even slightly acid. **Acid perms** have activators added to them and rely on heat to open the cuticle scales. They contain detergents to aid penetration of perm lotion into the cortex. **Tepid perms** are used with special hot clamps and require less heat than **hot perms**.

The **processing time** (length of time the perm lotion is left on) will vary according to:

1   The strength of ammonium thioglycollate (the stronger it is, the quicker it acts).
2   The pH (generally the higher the pH, the quicker the reaction).
3   The porosity of the hair (the more porous the hair the quicker the reaction).
4   The working temperature (heat speeds up chemical reactions, so the hotter it is, the quicker it will work).

Because of these variations it is important to check the manufacturer's instructions and to check the client's hair regularly (especially if heat is applied) to prevent over-processing which can severely damage the hair and cause hair breakage.

When a satisfactory curl has been obtained the perm lotion is rinsed from the hair with the curlers still in position.

The **second stage** is now carried out. In this so-called **neutralizing stage** the broken di-sulphide bonds are rebuilt in their new position along the polypeptide chains. This makes the new curled shape permanent. The chemical process which reforms the di-sulphide bonds is an **oxidation reaction** (not chemical neutralization) and is brought about by an oxidizing agent (hydrogen peroxide or sodium bromate). The oxidizing agent supplies oxygen which combines with the hydrogen to form water.

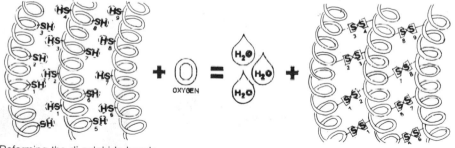

Reforming the di-sulphide bonds

Not all of the broken di-sulphide bonds will be reformed so that the number of di-sulphide linkages in hair is always reduced by perming. This will weaken the hair.

Hot perms

The hair must first be washed to remove grease and lacquer which would reduce penetration of the perm lotion into the cortex. The perm lotion (which contains a **reducing agent** such as **sodium** or **potassium** sulphate) is then added to the hair which is wound on to the curlers with some tension. Heat can now be applied by a variety of methods including electric heaters, hot metal clips, steam processing and exothermic pads. The di-sulphide bonds in keratin are broken partly by the chemical reaction of the reducing agent and partly by the action of the heat and the alkaline which produces a **hydrolysis reaction** (addition of water). The rebuilding of the linkages takes place at the same time as the breakdown process so there is no second stage reaction. The heated clips or pads remain in the hair until they are cool. They are then removed and the hair is rinsed.

After perm conditioning

Perming tends to leave the hair:
1   More porous (action of alkali).
2   Weaker and less elastic with a greater tendency to split (not all di-sulphide bonds are reformed).
3   With the cuticle scales open (action of alkali).

The use of an acid anti-oxidant (reducing agent) rinse such as **ascorbic acid** will neutralize any remaining alkaline, close the cuticle scales and stop the action of the oxidizing agent. Other conditioning creams may also be used.

PREPARATION

Discussion

Remember that this is a permanent wave, and is difficult to correct if the result is unsatisfactory.

If you have previously worked with the client's hair, ask if the temporary styling was satisfactory, and then decide with the client what would be the most suitable type of permanent wave. You should take into account the following factors about the client.

LIFE-STYLE   The client's life-style is very important, as busy people do not have as much time as they would like to dress their hair every day – perhaps the answer would be a natural look perm that is just washed and left to dry naturally? However, some people prefer a perfectly finished style and would not feel comfortable with this.

AGE   Age is also necessary to consider. For instance children's hair is very difficult to curl and using chemicals near their eyes can be hazardous. Mature clients often prefer a tighter result, which lasts longer, as retired people cannot always afford regular salon visits.

HEALTH   The client's health is also important as ill health can have detrimental affects on hair (see Chapter 5), and sometimes permanent waves can relax, becoming straight, in a very short period of time. Always ask clients if they are taking any medication from the doctor and if in doubt take a test-curl beforehand (see page 176).

New clients, as well as regular clients, must be questioned thoroughly about their permanent waving requirements, i.e. the finished style result, suitability for their needs (tightness or softness of curl), how long it will last, and of course the cost of the permanent wave. Remembering to include any hidden extras, e.g. cutting.

Keep regular records of all permanent waves done in the salon, and always refer to them.

Permanent Waving Record Card

Index No.

Name of client: Date of 1st Perm ....

Address: Colour treated or natural ....

                         If treated, product ....

Daytime Tel. No.   Texture ....

                         Condition ....

Date	Type of Lotion	Lotion Strength	Size of Curlers	Result Required	Development Time & Method	Special Notes	Neutralising Time & Method	Conditioner	Result Obtained	Stylist

Gowning up

Gown the client up with a protective gown, cape and towels to protect her from both permanent wave lotion and oxidizer solution.

Permanent wave lotion can be very damaging to your hands and fingernails, so always use protective gloves whilst applying it to the hair.

PERMANENT WAVE ANALYSIS

The following chart will help you to make an in-depth permanent waving analysis.

Permanent wave analysis Checklist

Name: Stylist:

Address: Date:

1 Client requirements: style/cut consideration:
                         type of curl:
2 Scalp condition
3 Hair thickness   6 Hair elasticity
4 Hair texture   7 Hair condition
5 Hair length   8 Hair porosity
9 Previous chemical treatments
10 Tests
11 Product used
     (a) strength   (b) rods used
     (c) winding method   (d) processing time
     (e) processing method   (f) oxidizing product used
     (g) oxidizing time
12 After treatment (e.g. conditioner)
13 Wet curl result
14 Dry curl result
15 Styling method
16 Homecare method
17 Homecare products sold
18 Special notes

Scalp

Always check the scalp for cuts and abrasions before perming as the lotion can be very damaging. Only small cuts and abrasions can be covered with collodion beforehand.

Hair

THICKNESS OR DENSITY Thick or abundant hair will need more lotion to be applied both during processing and during oxidization. Some lotions are available in individual bottles whilst others are dispensed from large containers, but between 30–60 cc is the usual amount.

Always discard unwanted lotion, never pour it back into the original container.

HAIR TEXTURE This means the coarseness or fineness of each individual hair. The amount of permanent wave lotion absorbed depends on the tightness of the cuticle scale, and some coarse hair can be porous whilst some fine hair can be non-porous and vice-versa. Negroid hair is particularly vulnerable so extra care should be taken.

HAIR LENGTH Special attention must be paid to longer hair which needs more permanent wave lotion. Remember to charge the client accordingly.

Not only must the length and ends be properly saturated with permanent wave lotion but the oxidizing solution must penetrate the ends for the process to be successful. Long hair often needs to be 'double neutralized'.

HAIR ELASTICITY This is known as testing the tensile strength to see if the hair can withstand a permanent wave process (see page 157). Hair that has been previously chemically treated is often over-stretchy and needs less tension when winding.

HAIR CONDITION If the hair is in poor condition from either chemical or mechanical damage (see page 152), then it may not be able to take a permanent wave. Frequent cutting helps, as does the use of a pre-perm conditioner.

POROSITY Damaged hair is often more porous and will absorb permanent wave lotion very quickly. Some hair is unevenly porous, e.g. on the ends, and may need a pre-perm lotion applied specifically to those areas to even out the porosity.

It is better to apply the permanent wave lotion after winding (post damping) for over-porous hair, and before winding (pre-damping) for non-porous hair.

Previous chemical treatments

Clients with hair colours or bleaches on their hair need special consideration. The hair will be more porous and needs either diluted permanent wave lotions or special strengths to suit that particular need – always read the manufacturer's instructions.

Occasionally, clients have used hair colour restorers on their hair. These are not always easy to detect and clients may not understand that they have chemically processed their hair. If in doubt take a test cutting.

TEST CUTTINGS Cut a small piece of hair (it is thickest at the back of the head), tie with cotton and complete an incompatibility test (see page 204).

It is the oxidizing solution that could react with the metallic salts on the hair.

Pre-test curls

If you are in any doubt about the hair being successfully permanently waved, then take a test curl. This will give you and your client confidence.

Either cut a small piece of hair and tie with cotton or proceed with a small section of hair on the head. Use the appropriate permanent wave lotion, the correct curler size and develop for the manufacturer's specified time, then oxidize as normal.

When the curl is dry it can be stored away safely or shown to the client immediately, and then the process can commence.

TECHNIQUES

Basic section wind

The following diagrams are for a basic nine section wind for a traditional hairstyle that is set with the aid of rollers.

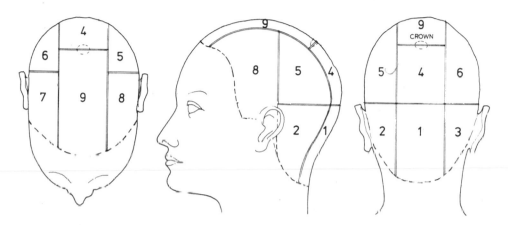

Winding normally begins at the nape area (see page 183 for sectioning).

Winding to achieve specific fashion results

Permanent wave winding can be both varied and exciting for both the hairdresser and the client. Fashion techniques may take a little longer to achieve, so remember to charge the client accordingly.

Many types of permanent wave curlers or rods are available. These

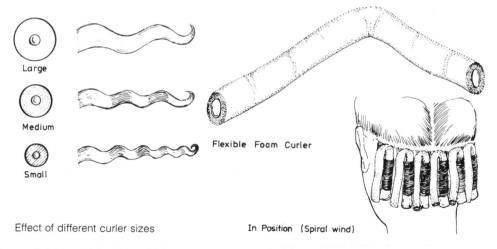

Effect of different curler sizes   In Position (Spiral wind)

curlers are available in many sizes. The smaller the curler – the tighter the curl. The larger the curler – the softer the curl. They are often colour coded so that the sizes can be easily recognized.

There are also flexible foam curlers with no rubbers to constrict the hair roots (rubber can permanently damage the hair if the curlers are too tight (see page 192). These can be used for both croquignole and spiral winding (see page 105).

Hair can even be shaped permanently to form a zig-zag effect by using special equipment.

Winding techniques can vary considerably to achieve many different looks. For example:

DIRECTIONAL WINDING

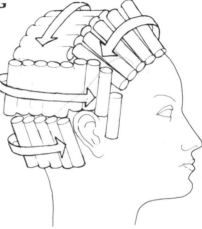

Directional Winding

The hair may be wound in the direction of the finished style.

BRICK WINDING

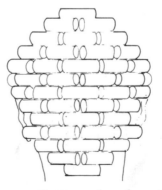

This technique ensures a more uniform curl and avoids partings in the finished result.

STACK WINDING OR PERIMETER CURL

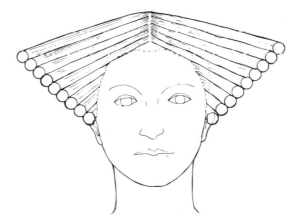

This type of wind will produce a straight effect on top and volume around the perimeter.

WEAVE WINDING

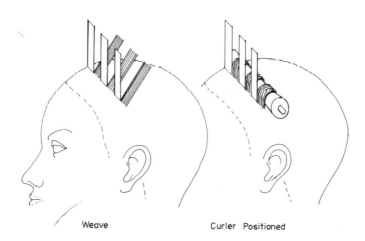

Weave   Curler Positioned

This is ideal when a spiky effect is needed, yet volume is needed on the roots. Normally large curlers are used.

MATERIALS

Barrier creams

These are heavy, thick creams which either are applied to the client, if she has a sensitive hairline, to prevent any lotion touching the skin, or may be used for protecting your hands if protective gloves are unacceptable.

Cotton wool

Cotton wool strips must be pre-dampened with warm water to prevent permanent wave lotion and oxidizer being absorbed into them during use. They are placed around the client's hairline to prevent any lotion from running into the eyes, ears or neck areas. If lotion has been absorbed into the cotton wool during processing, replace it immediately to prevent skin burns.

Cotton wool is also useful for absorbing excess moisture from the curlers before the oxidizer is applied.

Protective gloves

These must be worn whilst applying permanent wave lotion. If they are difficult to put on because your hands are damp, sprinkle some talcum powder inside them.

End papers

These are specially designed, absorbent papers which make winding easier and help to prevent 'fish hooks' (see page 105).

Permanent wave lotions

These are made for normal, resistant (non-porous), tinted, bleached and over-porous hair (acid perms are particularly good for damaged hair). Generally, more porous hair needs a weaker perm solution.

Manufacturers produce lotions specifically for fashion purposes and may combine them with special rods for that purpose. Pre-perm lotions are available for over-porous hair (see page 176).

Oxidant (neutralizer)

This is available either ready prepared in individual bottles or larger containers and is sometimes mixed or diluted. Read the manufacturer's instructions carefully.

EQUIPMENT

Accelerator

Permanent waves processed under an accelerator often require a plastic cap to prevent over-drying and scalp burns. (See page 44.)

Steamers

(See page 44.) Always check for safety (wires and plug tops) and clean regularly. Remember to check that the water container is maintained with an adequate amount of water before switching on. If the steamer is used for too long (over 15 minutes) during processing time, it may start to dilute the lotion and the perm will not process.

Applicator brushes, sponges and bottles

Both permanent wave lotions and oxidizing lotions may be applied by special bottles (fitted with applicator nozzles), brushes or sponges.
    Always rinse, clean and dry them after use. (See page 46.)

Bowls

Non-metallic bowls are used to contain either permanent wave lotion or oxidizing lotion. Bowls used for oxidizer (neutralizer) must be large enough to hold the lotion when it has been foamed up with a neutralizer sponge. (See page 46.)

Caps

Plastic caps are used on the client's hair during processing to preserve body heat and aid development. Disposable caps are often too large and need to be secured with a section clip. (See page 46.)

If other types of plastic cap are used (non-disposable), then they must be washed and dried thoroughly after use.

Curlers/rods

These are used for winding small meshes of hair and must be washed, rinsed and dried after use (see specific fashion results, page 177).

Measures

These are necessary for accurately measuring amounts of lotion. Always use a clean, dry measure, and check that the amount is correct, e.g. are you reading cc's or fluid oz's?

Pour the product carefully into the measure which should be on a level shelf, then bend down with your eyes level to the product in the measure to read it correctly (see page 53).

If the manufacturer's instructions direct you to add a capsule of activator (as with acid perms) then make sure it is thoroughly mixed in with the lotion at the right time (i.e. just *before* applying to the hair). Often applicator bottles with screw tops are supplied so that the activator and lotions can be mixed together by shaking.

Protective clothing

This is used to protect both you and your client from chemical splashes, and requires washing after use. Permanent wave lotions tend to decompose rubber and plastics if they are not rinsed off thoroughly.

Trolleys

See page 42. Always clean the trolley after use. In the same way that the metal tail of unprofessional pin tail combs can discolour (mauve/ brown) so can any straight setting pins that are left in the tray. If this discoloured lotion comes into contact with clients with light coloured hair, then their hair may become discoloured too!

METHODS

Shampooing

Select the appropriate shampoo for pre-perming, which may either be a clear soapless detergent with no additives or one specified by the manufacturer, and continue to shampoo in the correct manner (see Chapter 6).

Always check that the hair does not feel greasy before a perm, either from excessive natural oils or from pre-permanent wave conditioners or restructurants.

If the client's hair contains an excess of hairspray (often clients will hold hairspray too close to their hair and make the hair rigid), then use an appropriate de-lacquer shampoo (see page 85).

Sectioning

Comb the hair thoroughly to remove tangles (see page 87), then towel dry the hair to prevent the lotions from being diluted.

The traditional nine section method of winding, including the sizes of the sub-sections, is described on page 177 (basic section wind).

Start at the front hairline and make sure that Section One is in the centre, and parallel.

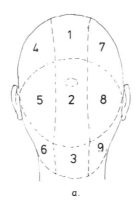

a.

Always measure the size of the sections against the length of the curler – the section should be just a little smaller.

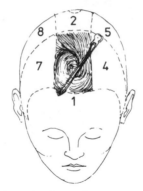

Section One will end just before the crown area. Secure each section, with either a section clip or butterfly clip, neatly on its own base. Continue with section two which ends at the top of the ear, then complete section three down to the nape. Check that sections one, two and three are in the centre of the head, not lop-sided.

Continue with section four, measuring both the top and bottom of the section with the curler. To complete sections five and six, section from the top of section three across to the top of the ear, level with the bottom of section four.

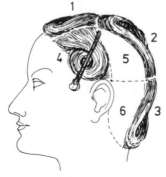

Repeat sections four, five and six on the opposite side of the head to complete sections seven, eight and nine.

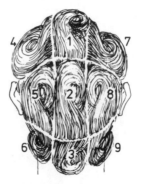

Sectioning is very important as it enables you to work quickly and methodically from section to section and see the size of the curlers used previously.

Winding

SUB-SECTIONING   The length of the curlers decides the section size, but the depth or width of the curler decides the size of the sub-section. Each sub-section must be parallel or uneven winding will result.

Once the hair has been sub-sectioned the mesh of hair is combed smoothly away from the head at a 90° angle.

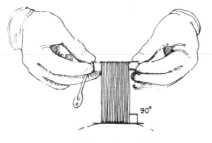

Winding hair at 90°

WINDING THE CURLERS   Use a pin tail comb and start to wind the ends around the curler, using end papers if necessary to prevent 'fish hooks' (see page 105). Wind without undue tension on the hair.

SITTING CURLERS ON THEIR BASE   Keep the curler parallel to the head whilst winding, or else the curler will not sit properly on the sub-section.

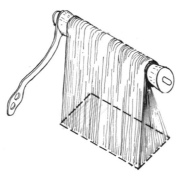

Curler parallel to base

As client's heads are round (not square) and the curlers are straight, perfect winding is difficult to achieve without practice.

Not all curlers are wound to the root, winding can vary according to different techniques (see page 179, Stack winding).

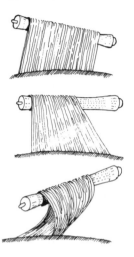

Non-parallel winding

FASTENING THE CURLERS   Perm curlers with rubber attached to the ends must be fastened securely but without stress or tension on the hair root. Always check that the rubbers are not twisted before securing them.

If there is tension on the hair roots from the rubbers being too tight then extensive damage can be caused (see page 192).

Manufacturers supply plastic strips which can be inserted across the top of the curlers and under the rubbers to keep the curlers in place and prevent them from marking the hair.

Lotioning the hair

PRE-DAMPING   This is when the hair is lotioned after sectioning, and during sub-sectioning. This technique is often used for resistant hair (non-porous).

POST-DAMPING   This is when the lotion is applied after winding has been completed, and applicator bottles fitted with special nozzles are often used.

SAFE PRACTICES

Applying perm lotion can be very dangerous, as it can so easily run into the client's eyes. If this does happen, rinse immediately with cold water from a tap or eye-wash bottle until the client says that the stinging has stopped.

Always take extra precautions by using a strip of dampened cotton wool around the hairline and holding a piece of cotton wool near the applicator bottle (if used) during lotioning to absorb any excess.

NB Many manufacturers' individual bottles of permanent wave lotion and neutralizer look very similar! To prevent applying the wrong lotion at the wrong time get the oxidizer out of the dispensary only at the time of neutralizing.

Processing

MANUFACTURER'S INSTRUCTIONS Always read and follow the manufacturers' instructions for processing. Sometimes they are printed on leaflets inside the carton and often are printed on the carton itself.

Try to attend as many manufacturers' courses as possible to see the products in use for yourself. Many manufacturers have specialist technicians who will come to the salon to explain their products.

It is important to check your product knowledge regularly as new products and their uses are constantly being developed to meet the needs of hairdressing/perming fashions.

TESTING THE CURL STRENGTH Once the lotion has been applied, it is important to take test curls at frequent intervals – especially with over-porous hair which will process very quickly.

Some permanent waves are processed without heat, just a plastic cap, whilst others must be processed with heat or they will not work!

It is very important not to leave your client unattended at this stage, and you must check the processing regularly.

The temperature of the salon also makes a difference. Perms will process quicker on warm days than on cold ones. Check also that your client is not sitting near a draught from an open door or window, as one side of the hair may process more quickly than the other!

CHECKING THE TEST CURL IS READY FOR OXIDATION

This process takes a lot of practice and experience, so watch closely when senior staff are doing it.

Always take test curls on different areas of the head, remember one area may be ready before another. If this has happened, then dilute the area which has taken with water to slow down the processing.

Method

1 Undo the rubber fastener, at one end of the curler.
2 Unwind the curler 1½ turns, without letting the hair unravel completely. Hold the hair firmly with both thumbs touching the curler.
3 Push the hair towards the scalp allowing it to relax into an 'S' shaped movement. **Do not pull the hair** – remember it is in a very fragile state.
4 When the size of the 'S' shape corresponds to the size of the curler, the processing time can be stopped.

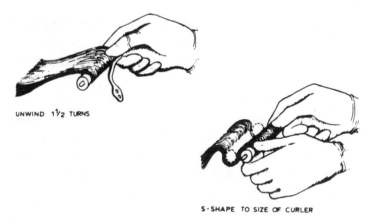

UNWIND 1½ TURNS

S-SHAPE TO SIZE OF CURLER

Taking a test curl

Oxidizing

CHOOSING THE CORRECT OXIDIZER Each permanent wave lotion has its own special oxidizing solution. Try to use one made by the same manufacturer, and always check the manufacturer's instructions. Some may give a special mixing or application procedure (they do not all foam up), whilst others may need special strengths for over-porous hair.

RINSING   Once the processing is complete, take the client to the washbasin and check that he or she is comfortable.

Apply a dampened strip of cotton wool to the hairline and proceed to rinse the curlers using as hot a water temperature as the client can comfortably bear – remember to ask! Use your free hand to cup the water over the curlers and back down into the washbasin.

Continue rinsing until all the chemical wave solution has been removed from the hair (about five minutes).

BLOTTING THE CURLERS   All excess water must now be removed before the oxidizing solution is applied, or it will not work!

You may either use a dry absorbent towel or a wad of cotton wool, pressed carefully into the curlers so as not to disturb them. Remember the hair is still very soft and fragile.

Up to two fluid ounces of water can be removed – so make sure you do it properly.

APPLYING THE OXIDIZER   Check that you have the correct oxidizing solution and the correct equipment to apply it. Some oxidizers are applied by foaming the lotion in a large bowl with a neutralizer sponge; other lotions are applied to the hair, then foamed up with the sponge on the curlers. Others are poured directly from a bottle with a special applicator nozzle.

TIMING   Each manufacturer will specify a different length of time to leave the oxidizing solution on (five minutes is the average time).

However, this is a messy process, and busy salons may need the washbasin for another client. In this case a drip tray is placed around the client's neck to catch any excess lotion, whilst she is seated at a dressing position.

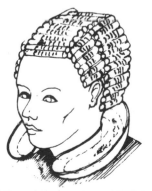

Drip tray in use

To oxidize long hair properly, a technique called **double neutralizing** is used. The oxidizer is left for the normal time, then each curler is unwound individually and oxidizer is applied to the lengths of hair. The curler is then wound back up to the scalp and refastened. The oxidizer is then left for another five minutes. This technique will help to prevent the curl from relaxing and the hair becoming straight.

REMOVAL OF CURLERS When the oxidization is complete, each curler is gently removed without exerting any undue tension on the hair. Always start removing the curlers from underneath the nape area if using a backwash, and work methodically through each wound section.

If any oxidizer is left over, it cannot be used again once it has been exposed to the air, so apply it to the hair lengths now.

RINSING OUT THE OXIDIZER Once all the curlers have been removed, rinse the hair thoroughly with warm water.

CONDITIONING Some manufacturers specify their own after-perm conditioner, so check the instructions.

It is normal procedure to apply a conditioner, and an **anti-oxidant**, such as ascorbic acid, is particularly good. The client's scalp may be tender after a permanent wave, so make sure you do not pull the hair unnecessarily whilst combing the conditioner through the hair lengths.

If a restructurant is to be applied (for over-porous hair), then towel dry the hair before you apply it. Remember many restructurants are not rinsed out.

RECORD CARDS The perming record card is normally completed at this stage, before styling, and should then be filed away.

UNDESIRABLE EFFECTS FOLLOWING PERMING

Fault	Causes
Overprocessing (the hair is frizzy when wet and looks straight when dry)	1 Incorrect analysis (see page 174). too strong permanent wave lotion used (see page 180). 2 Incorrect processing time (see page 171). and not testing the curl development properly (see page 188). 3 Choosing the incorrect permanent wave lotioning technique, i.e. pre-or post-dampening (see page 186). 4 Using too much heat during processing (see page 171).
Underprocessing (the perm is not curly enough)	1 Incorrect analysis (see page 174). 2 Incorrectly shampooed hair – either naturally greasy hair or conditioner/restructurants forming a barrier to the permanent wave lotion (see page 183). 3 Insufficient permanent wave lotion applied, or too weak lotion used. 4 Processing time too short and no allowance made for cold salon conditions (see page 187). 5 Incorrect oxidizing, i.e. poor blotting after rinsing, insufficient lotion applied and insufficient timing (see page 189).
Failure to achieve intended curl POOR WINDING RESULT	1 Incorrect selection of curlers or winding equipment – either too large, too small or too few curlers. 2 Incorrect winding technique for hair length (see page 178). Poor winding. 'Fish Hooks' (see page 185) must be cut off.

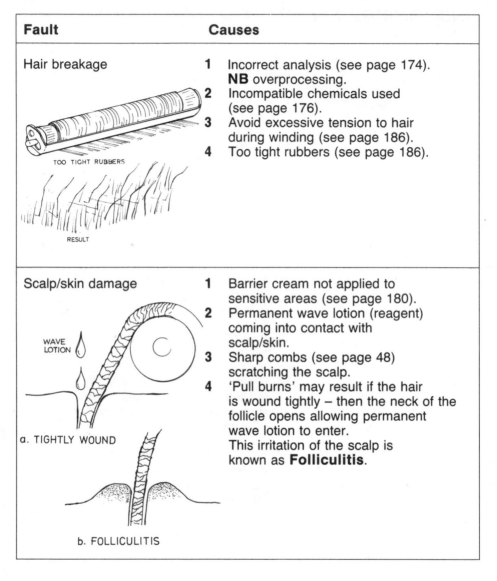

Fault	Causes
Hair breakage	1 Incorrect analysis (see page 174). **NB** overprocessing.
	2 Incompatible chemicals used (see page 176).
	3 Avoid excessive tension to hair during winding (see page 186).
	4 Too tight rubbers (see page 186).
Scalp/skin damage	1 Barrier cream not applied to sensitive areas (see page 180).
	2 Permanent wave lotion (reagent) coming into contact with scalp/skin.
	3 Sharp combs (see page 48) scratching the scalp.
	4 'Pull burns' may result if the hair is wound tightly – then the neck of the follicle opens allowing permanent wave lotion to enter. This irritation of the scalp is known as **Folliculitis**.

HAIR STRAIGHTENING

Hair may be straightened or relaxed either **temporarily** (see Chapter 7) or **permanently**.

Permanent hair straightening

This is a highly skilled process. The chemicals used are the same as those used in perming but much stronger and great care must be taken to guard against damaging the hair. Since the cream or lotion may come into contact with the scalp, extra care must be taken when examining for skin conditions beforehand.

PERMANENT HAIR STRAIGHTENING ANALYSIS CHECKLIST

Name:

Address: Stylist:

Tel. No.   Date:

1 Client requirements } style/cut consideration
                        } type of curl
2 Scalp condition
3 Hair thickness
4 Hair texture
5 Hair length
6 Hair elasticity
7 Hair condition
8 Hair porosity
9 Previous chemical treatments
10 Tests
11 Product used
   (a) strength   (e) processing method
   (b) rods used   (f) oxidizing
   (c) winding method   (g) oxidizing time
   (d) processing time
12 After treatment (e.g. conditioner):
13 Wet curl result
14 Dry curl result
15 Styling methods
16 Homecare method
17 Homecare products sold
18 Special notes

Special precautions

You should follow these precautions:

1 Always wear protective gloves.
2 Never use metal tools (i.e. non-anodized steel).
3 When applying a straightener to a regrowth, **do not overlap** onto the previously straightened hair. Do not overprocess – the cream will act as a **depilatory** (hair remover).

Method

You should follow these procedures:

1 Always use a soapless shampoo and towel dry.
2 Disentangle the hair – a rinse is occasionally supplied.
3 Section the hair, dividing it into four sections.

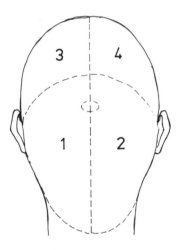

Sections for straightening

4 Apply cream to the front hairline first, then the nape. Use a wide toothed comb to stretch the hair as flat as possible.
5 Process the hair following the manufacturer's directions and test for lack of wave formation.
6 Remove cream from the hair using a backwash basin and rinse thoroughly, combing the hair straight.
7 Neutralize the hair – mix oxidizer and saturate the hair. Comb hair straight continuously for five minutes.
8 Complete the procedure by applying conditioner and rinse and set.

Chemistry

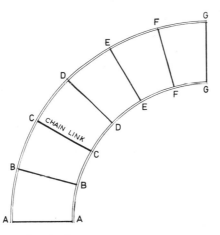

Normal curly shape

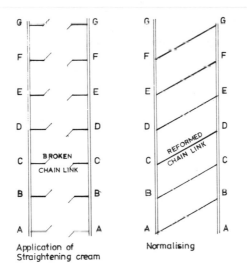

Application of   Normalising
Straightening cream

The chemical reaction is basically the same as that for cold permanent waving. However, instead of the hair being wound onto small rollers during the first stage of perming, it is either wound onto large diameter rollers or the perm lotion is combed through the hair. Hair straightening lotions tend to contain a greater concentration of ammonium thioglycollate and may be of a higher pH (pH10), than normal perm lotions. Modern chemical straighteners, like the acid and tepid perms, are much milder than this and use the reducing agents sodium or ammonium bisulphite and heat to speed up the chemical reaction of breaking the di-sulphide bonds.

A comparison between permanently straightening and waving hair

Permanently straightening	Permanently waving

Perm lotion
pH range 10–14
	Perm lotion
	pH range
	    6–7.5 acid permanent waves
	    9–9.5 alkali permanent waves

Cream or jelly	Liquid
Chemical usually comes into contact with the scalp.	Lotions should not come into contact with the scalp.
Combed flat or wound on very large curlers.	Wound on curlers.
Usually started at front hairline.	Usually started in the nape area.
Test for processing by lack of wave formation.	Test for processing by definite wave formation.

MULTIPLE CHOICE QUESTIONS

1   the pH of an ordinary cold permanent wave lotion is approximately:
    (a) 4–5   (c) 6–8
    (b) 9–10   (d) 12–13

2   In which part of the hair do the chemical processes involved in perming take place:
    (a) cuticle
    (b) cortex
    (c) medulla
    (d) dermal papilla

3   An increase in temperature will speed up the action of perm lotion because higher temperatures:
    (a) increase the rate of evaporation
    (b) close the cuticle scales
    (c) decrease the rate of chemical reactions
    (d) increase the rate of chemical reactions

4   The reducing agent in perm lotion is:
    (a) hydrogen peroxide
    (b) ammonium hydroxide
    (c) ammonium thioglycollate
    (d) citric acid

5   The chemical bonds in keratin which are most affected by perm lotion are the:
    (a) peptide bonds
    (b) hydrogen bonds
    (c) disulphide bonds
    (d) oxidizing bonds

6   The chemical process which occurs in the second stage of cold permanent waving is:
    (a) neutralization
    (b) oxidation
    (c) reduction
    (d) hydrogenation

7   Test curls are taken to determine:
    (a) lotion strength and timing
    (b) tensile strength of hair
    (c) the condition of the cuticle
    (d) the degree of curl

8   The second or 'neutralizer' stage of the permanent wave reaction
     has the effect of:
     (a)   opening the cuticle scales
     (b)   relaxing the curl
     (c)   fixing the curl
     (d)   closing the cuticle scale

9   An oxidizing agent which may be used in the 'neutralizer' stage
     of permanent waving is:
     (a)   sodium bromate
     (b)   sodium hydroxide
     (c)   sodium chloride
     (d)   sodium thioglycollate

10   Ascorbic acid may be used as:
     (a)   an oxidizing agent
     (b)   a hydrolysing agent
     (c)   an anti-static rinse
     (d)   an after-perm conditioning rinse

11   The result of permanent wave lotion entering the hair follicles
     during lotioning is:
     (a)   greater lift at the roots
     (b)   psoriasis
     (c)   folliculitis and pull burns
     (d)   increased rate of hair growth

12   Permanent hair straighteners will act as depilatories if the pH is:
     (a)   10–14   (c)   4–5
     (b)   9–10   (d)   1–2

13   End papers are used to:
     (a)   speed up processing time
     (b)   help spread perm lotion
     (c)   prevent perm lotion touching curler
     (d)   make winding easier

14   One cause of *Trichorrhexis nodosa* is:
     (a)   loss of di-sulphide bonds during permanent waving
     (b)   too tight permanent wave rubbers
     (c)   too strong perm lotion
     (d)   too high tension when winding

15   The type of shampoo used before perming is:
     (a)   medicated   (c)   anti-oxy
     (b)   conditioning   (d)   soapless with no additives

11
PERMANENT OXIDATION TINTING

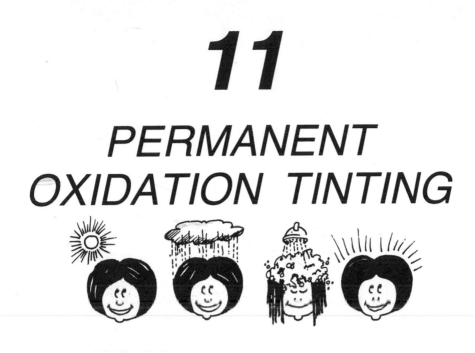

NATURAL HAIR COLOUR

Natural pigments

Natural pigments are found in the hair cortex. They are produced by special cells called melanocytes. There are three types of pigment:

Melanin	**Pheomelanin**	**Trichosiderin**
(brown/black)	(red/yellow)	(red)

Natural hair colour depends on the types of pigments present (usually a mixture) and the quantity of pigments.

Hair that has never been artificially coloured is known as **virgin** hair.

To change the colour of hair, new pigments are added, either to the hair cortex or to the surface of the hair. Hair colour can also be changed by bleaching.

Note: Before you begin any hair colouring, always remember to protect your client's clothing, yourself and your clothing.

HAIR COLOURANTS

Types of colourant

Colourants may be **temporary** (washes out during first wash), **semi-permanent** (6-8 washes), **quasi-permanent** (10-12 washes), or **permanent**. Colourants may also be classified according to their chemical composition.

Natural vegetable dyes	Metallic dyes	Synthetic dyes
e.g. Camomile (temporary) Henna (permanent)	e.g. Hair colour restorers (permanent)	*Permanent tints* e.g. 'Para' dyes or oxidation dyes (mixed with hydrogen peroxide
		Semi-permanent tints e.g. Nitro dyes and anthraquinone dyes
		Quasi-permanent tints A mixture of oxidation and semi-permanent dyes
		Temporary tints e.g. direct or azo dyes and basic dyes

Non permanent dyes are dealt with in Chapter 13.

PERMANENT TINTS

Permanent tints are used to create exciting colour changes by means of a **chemical oxidation process** (see page 210).

Types

They are available as creams, gels and cream/gel mixtures.

All types are mixed in equal parts with hydrogen peroxide. The chemical reaction between the dye and the hydrogen peroxide is an oxidation reaction. They are therefore known as **oxidation tints.**

NB Secure all tops and lids of any unused dye to prevent premature oxidation.

Uses

1   To add colour tone, darken hair colours and lighten hair colours.
2   To cover white hair, a full head, or re-growth colour.
3   To neutralize unwanted tones in hair, e.g. yellow, brassy colours.
4   For highlights (use a highlifting tint), low lights or fashion colouring.

Skin tests

Skin tests are used to test for allergic reactions to permanent colours (i.e. 'para' dyes). The dyes are toxic and can cause contact dermatitis (eczema).

Predisposition
Sabouraud-Rousseau   } are alternative names for a skin test
Patch tests

FREQUENCY   Skin tests must be carried out before each application of dye (usually 24-48 hours before). A positive reaction (redness, blistering, itching, etc.) means that the client must have no further exposure to the 'para' dye.

Method

1   Clean a small sensitive area of skin (either behind the ear or in the crook of the elbow) with cotton wool and surgical spirit.
2   Mix a small volume of equal quantities of the darkest tone colour plus 20 vol. (6%) peroxide and carefully apply to the area. Allow to dry.
3   Cover with collodian and allow to dry.
4   Ask the client to leave the patch test for 24-48 hours. If there is any redness, soreness, itching or swelling, then the client must inform the salon that he/she has had a positive reaction and is allergic to the dye.

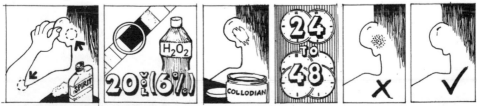

5 A record card must be completed, stating the client's name and address and the date of the skin test.

HAIR COLOUR RECORD CARD

Name of Client: _____ Natural hair colour _____

Address: _____ Texture _____

_____ Condition _____

Tel. No. _____

Skin test   Date: Name of operator:

Record of application

Date	Type	Colour	Hydrogen peroxide	Development		Aplication special notes	Comb through	After treat-ment	Result		Stylist
				Method	Time				Req'd	Obt'd	

HAIR COLOUR ANALYSIS

For a more in-depth analysis the following chart may be a useful guide.

Hair colour analysis checklist

Name:

Address: Stylist:

Tel. No.   Date:

Scalp

1 Skin test
2 Scalp analysis
3 Strand test

Hair

1 Natural base (i.e. natural depth and tone)
2 Hair condition
3 Tensile strength
4 Porosity
5 Hair texture
6 Hair length
7 Abundance
8 Percentage of white hair and distribution
9 Previous chemical treatments
10 Client's choice of colour
11 Target shade and product used
12 Peroxide strength and type used
13 Method of application (including comb through)
14 Development time and equipment used
15 After treatment
16 Result obtained
17 Special notes

Skin

1 Skin tone

Client

1 Personality and life-style
2 Approximate age
3 Special notes
4 Client preference
5 Homecare advice

Precautions

Test cuttings or **strand tests** (i.e. a small sample of hair secured with cotton) are taken if there is any doubt about chemicals used previously on the hair, i.e. metallic dyes (hair colour restorers). The metal salts found in hair colour restorers will react violently with hydrogen peroxide and produce intense heat which can burn and cause hair breakage (see page 212).

Mix 1 part ammonium hydroxide plus 30 parts 20 vol. (6%) hydrogen peroxide. If incompatible, steam and breakage will occur.

Test cuttings are also useful to assess the resultant colour on the hair for clients who are undecided when choosing the colour. Mix the proposed colour with the chosen strength of peroxide and leave to develop for time and a half (to allow for lack of body heat).

Remember to protect the client with a gown, shoulder cape, towels, tissues and, if necessary, barrier cream around the hairline (see page 180).

Examination of scalp

Check the scalp for any inflammations, cuts or abrasions and coat small abrasions with collodian.

Examination of hair

HAIR POROSITY Hair that is more porous due to perming, highlights, mechanical damage or simply because it is long, will absorb colour more quickly in some areas and an uneven colour will result. Also, tint will fade more quickly on porous hair.

The type of hair, whether it is Caucasian, Negroid or Asian (see page 71), will also affect the porosity. Often Negroid hair tends to be non-porous and difficult to tint.

HAIR TEXTURE You should note whether the individual hairs are coarse or fine and then the general abundance of hair on the head. Hair dyes generally appear to give a darker tone when the hair is fine and abundant. Very coarse hair may need a cream tint.

NATURAL HAIR COLOUR You should note the natural (base) shade, i.e. how light or dark it is compared to the tone, does it appear red, copper or ashen? Note if there are any white hairs present (there is no such thing as grey hair, it is white hair mixed with the natural colour). If any white hair is present remember the colour will show up more strongly e.g. red will appear much brighter. Tints may be used not only to colour white hair, but to darken, lighten or add stronger tones (e.g. more red, copper or ash).

Examination of skin tone/colour

Generally younger clients have fuller, plumper skin without lines and wrinkles. Older clients' skins not only change shape and texture but also lose colour tone. Very few older people have naturally rosy cheeks. It is often broken veins or cosmetic make-up (see page 31) that you see. Therefore young people can colour their hair most colours (but avoid red with a florid complexion), and look good.

Dark or ashen colours can be very ageing on older clients — they may wish to look younger   but their natural colour when they were young does not always suit them as they become older!

DEPTH AND TONE Most manufacturers use the ICC (International Colouring Code) numbering system for choosing colours.

◄──────────────── **Tone** ────────────────►

Tone \ Depth	Basic Shades	.1 (Blue) Ash	.2 (Violet) Mauve Ash	.3 (Yellow) Gold	.4 (Orange) Warm	.5/.6 (Red) Red	(Green) Matt Concentrate Colour
10 Lightest blonde							
9 Very light blonde		e.g. very light ash blonde 9.1					
8 Light blonde							
7 Blonde				e.g. golden blonde 7.3			
6 Dark blonde							
5 Light brown					e.g. light warm brown 5.4		
4 Brown							
3 Dark brown							
2 Very dark brown							
1 Black							

HOW LIGHT ↑ / HOW DARK ↓

EQUIPMENT

Gloves

Always wear gloves when tinting to prevent skin staining and dye dermatitis.

Applicators

Tints may be applied with either a tint brush (see page 46) or by an applicator bottle or gun fixed with a special nozzle. Tint brushes are normally used.

METHODS AND TECHNIQUES

Shampooing prior to tinting

This is not normally necessary, only in the case of excess grease or hairspray on the hair. Dry the hair completely before starting.

Mixing

HYDROGEN PEROXIDE The strength of hydrogen peroxide solution may be measured as percentage strength (%) or volume strength (vol.).

10 vol. or 3% — used to add weak colour (i.e. bleach toners)
20 vol. or 6% — used to add colour (i.e. for most tinting purposes)
30 vol. or 9% — used to lighten the colour of the base shade (see Chapter 12)
40 vol. or 12% — used for highlights and not generally considered suitable for scalp contact

See Chapter 12, pages 227–229 for details of hydrogen peroxide storage, strength and dilution.

TINT QUANTITIES Always check the manufacturer's instructions, but tint is generally mixed in equal quantities. Half a tube is normally sufficient for a regrowth, or a whole tube for a virgin head, very thick hair or a comb through application.

Sectioning

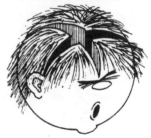

Divide hair into equal sections (usually four).

Regrowth application

(See diagram page 231.)
   Apply tint to the roots; use 6 mm partings. Do not overlap. If the ends are faded, comb through using the remaining tint and warm water and apply to 50 mm partings. Faded ends may be due to perming or atmospheric conditions, e.g. strong sunlight.

Virgin head application

To darken or lighten virgin hair apply to the middle lengths and ends first using 6 mm partings and to the roots last, to allow for the effects of body heat which will speed up the processing time (see page 230).

Checking tint application

Ensure that the hair is sufficiently loosened to allow circulation of air.
   Check the application by sectioning in the opposite direction, and re-applying to any uncovered areas. Assess whether or not the ends need to be combed through. This is not necessary every time. Remove any tint that may stain the skin at this stage. Remember to check that your client is comfortable.

Developing

Consult the manufacturer's directions; does it need heat or not? How long should it be left before checking? (The average time is 30 minutes.) Remember if heat is used (normally an accelerator) the development time is halved. Heat accelerates chemical reactions — but beware of over-processing which can damage the hair.

Checking the colour development

Remove some of the colour from the roots and the ends with damp cotton wool and compare the two colours. If they are of the required shade remove the colour.

Removal of the hair-colourant

One or two shampoos of a mild type are generally necessary and all
tint skin stains should be removed at the basin. An anti-oxidant (a
reducing agent) and acid rinse e.g. ascorbic acid are generally applied
to prevent the tint from oxidizing any further and to seal the colour.

Complete the Client Record Card at this stage. (See page 202.)

Multi-colours and part head colours

Style the hair first and study the areas where the colour will appear,
for instance a large amount of strong colour at the back of the head
may be completely covered by the rest of the hair when it has been
styled.

There are many techniques which can create exciting and varied
results such as highlights, lowlights, and block coloration.

Foil, self-adhesive strips and wrapping film will all separate the
colours from each other and prevent seepage.

Make sure that the sub-sections are appropriate to the amount of
hair needing to be coloured and the size of the material used, i.e.
width of the foil

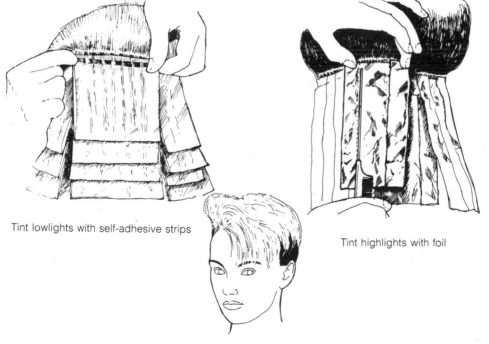

Tint lowlights with self-adhesive strips

Tint highlights with foil

Block colouration

These processes do take time to achieve, so remember to re-mix the tint every 30-40 minutes and to discard the unused amount.

CHEMICAL ACTION OF OXIDATION DYES

Oxidation dyes are small molecule dyes which are mixed with hydrogen peroxide. The oxygen from the hydrogen peroxide and the dye molecule link together inside the hair shaft to form larger molecules that cannot escape. This is an **oxidation reaction.** The tint is alkaline which swells the normally acid hair and opens the cuticle scale to aid penetration of the dye and hydrogen peroxide. The oxidized dye remains permanently inside the hair shaft because its now large molecules cannot escape and they do not dissolve in water. An anti-oxidant, e.g. ascorbic acid, is then applied, to prevent further hydrogen peroxide action and to help close down the cuticle scales (because it is also acidic in nature).

Oxidation dyes are also known as:

'Para dyes'
aromatic diamines (e.g. para-phenylene diamine,
para-toluenediamine)
analine derivatives

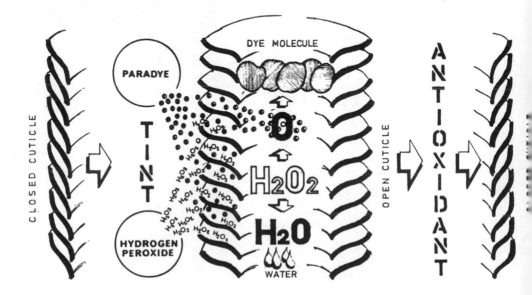

VEGETABLE DYES

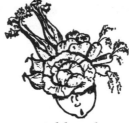

Henna

This is the most widely known vegetable colourant. It originated from the privet plant (*Lawsone*) which grows throughout Asia and Northern Africa. It is widely known for its conditioning properties.

USES It gives added tone, i.e. red or copper to hair, and the colour varies according to the client's natural colour, the henna colour and the timing.

APPLICATION The powder must be mixed to a smooth paste with very hot water and kept hot during the application (by using a double saucepan). The paste is applied all over the hair (it is very difficult and messy to apply) and covered with a plastic cap whilst developing with heat. It may be developed for any length of time according to the strength of colour required. Removal is by rinsing thoroughly, then shampooing.

CHEMISTRY Henna is a natural oxidation dye. The final permanent colour develops over several days as the dye molecules are slowly oxidized by oxygen in the air (hydrogen peroxide is not used). For this reason it is known as a **progressive dye.**

Vegetable/metallic dyes

Minerals or metallic salts were at one time added to Henna and known as compound Henna. This was to increase the colour range of pure Henna producing shades of blonde, light brown, mid-brown, brown, dark brown and black.

Metallic dyes

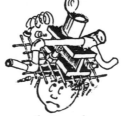

These are generally sold in shops as 'hair colour restorers' and contain metallic salts (black lead sulphide) which develop colour gradually over a period of time. They are difficult to recognize on a client's hair but can give the hair a 'greenish' shine and make the hair feel rather hard and rough. If a permanent wave neutralizer, an oxidation tint or any bleach (these all contain hydrogen peroxide) is used on hair that has been treated with 'colour restorer' or any metallic dye, then a green colour, steam and breakage may occur! (See page 204.)

CHEMISTRY Metallic dyes are also known as reduction, mineral, sulphide and progressive dyes. They consist of metal salts, e.g. lead acetate, silver nitrate, copper sulphate.

REDUCTION AND REMOVAL OF COLOURANTS

Removal of unwanted colour — colour cancellation

If tinting the hair results in the development of unwanted colours, this may be corrected by the addition of a small quantity of a further pigment which absorbs the offending complementary colour. For example, unwanted green can be absorbed by red, unwanted orange can be absorbed by blue, etc.

The colour triangle illustrates this **colour cancellation.** Any colour shown can be cancelled by the addition of small quantities of the opposite colour.

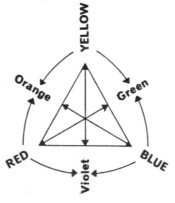

Red, yellow and blue are known as primary colours of pigments. Orange, violet and green are known as secondary colours of pigments.

Prepigmentation When colouring bleached hair back to natural brown, a red or copper pigment must be added or the hair colour will be green.

Removal of unwanted colour — colour reducers

These are made by hair-colouring companies to remove oxidation tints from hair (rather than using bleach).

They may be mixed with either water or peroxide according to the desired result. Always check the manufacturer's instructions for mixing, application method and development time as this is a highly skilled process.

Chemistry Colour reducers are chemically either:

Sodium bisulphite or
Sodium formaldehyde sulphoxylate

They break down the large dye molecules (produced by mixing 'para' tint and hydrogen peroxide) into small dye molecules which are then washed out of the hair, i.e. they reverse the dyeing process.

UNDESIRABLE EFFECTS FOLLOWING PERMANENT HAIR COLOURING

Fault	Reason	Treatment
Insufficient coverage	1 Strong white hair. 2 Peroxide strength weakened. 3 Make-up around the hairline.	1 Pre-soften with 10 vol. peroxide then apply tint and peroxide. 2 Re-apply with fresh tint and peroxide. 3 Clean with spirit and reapply tint.

Continued on page 214

Fault	Reason	Treatment
Too light	1 Insufficient time on the comb through. 2 Porous hair — either over permed or over tinted and will not hold the colour.	1 Lengthen the development time/use the accelerator. 2 Try a darker shade or use colour rinses between shampoos.
Too dark	1 Over porous hair. 2 Too many comb throughs. 3 Hair is finer around the front hairline. NB If time allows take a test cutting to determine the product strength and timing.	Either use colour reducers or equal parts weak paste bleach, peroxide and shampoo or highlifting tint.
Patchy result	Unevenly porous hair.	Cut off very porous ends.
Too matt (green)	Insufficient red pigment in hair.	Apply a red colour.
Too red	Insufficient brown.	Apply a matt colour (green).
Too orange	Insufficient black/brown pigment in hair.	Apply a blue based ash colour.
Too yellow	Insufficient black/brown pigment in hair.	Apply a violet based ash colour.

SALON LIGHTING

Light

Light is a form of energy which is absorbed by the eyes for vision. Pure white light as obtained from sunlight consists of a mixture of all the colours of the rainbow: red, orange, yellow, green, blue, indigo, violet. This is known as a spectrum. Each colour represents a different wavelength of light.

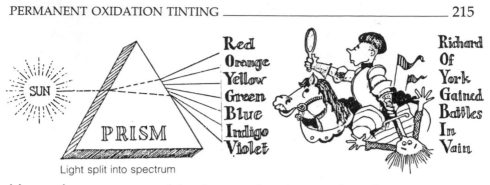

Red
Orange
Yellow
Green
Blue
Indigo
Violet

Richard
Of
York
Gained
Battles
In
Vain

Light split into spectrum

How do we see objects as having colour?

Coloured objects contain **pigments**. When white light shines upon pigments, certain colours (wavelengths of light) are absorbed by them. The rest of the colours are reflected back. We see only the colours that are reflected, e.g. a red object absorbs all the colours of the spectrum except red which is reflected. Therefore we see this object as red. A white object does not absorb any of the colours, all are reflected back and therefore we see white. A black object absorbs all the colours and reflects none. We see that object as black, i.e. an absence of colour.

The colour of hair is seen in the same way, the hair pigment absorbs one or more of the colours of the spectrum and reflects the remainder. We see only those colours which are reflected.

What factors affect the colours we see?

The type (or colour) of light shining on the object will affect the colour we see. We will see the 'real' colour only in pure white light (e.g. natural daylight). Artificially produced light is not pure white and will therefore affect the colours that we see.

Types of lighting available

The correct salon lighting is vital when hairdressing. The aim is to provide general good diffused light without glare, with additional lighting as necessary in working areas.

FLUORESCENT TUBES   The best system for general salon lighting is by fluorescent tubes. Different types of tubes give different qualities of light. Warm white tubes should be used for salon work since they provide light which is very similar to daylight (therefore good for colour work). Fluorescent tubes are more expensive to install than filament lamps, but they are much cheaper to run. Ash or blue fluorescent lights will neutralize warm or red colours.

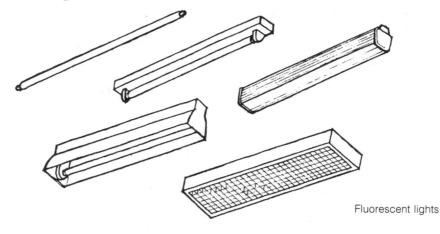

Fluorescent lights

FILAMENT LAMPS   These may be used as pearlised bulbs with a lamp shade to provide diffused light or as spot lights. All filament lamps give a reddish-yellow light, containing less blue and green than daylight. Thus blue and green shades appear darker and red brighter than in daylight.

Bare electric bulbs and spotlights can add warmth to hair colour and sometimes neutralize ash tones.

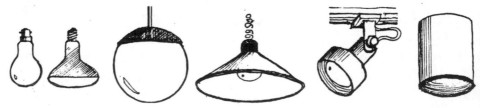

Effect of wall and ceiling colour

Wall and ceiling colourings will affect the quality of light in the salon. For instance red walls will reflect only red light and will therefore affect the apparent hair colour, i.e. reds will look brighter. Blue walls will reflect only blue, thus reds will look darker, etc. Look at the walls next to the client, green and blue walls will neutralize warm hair colours, whereas red and pink walls will make the same warm hair colours stronger. Coloured walls and ceiling will also absorb light and make the salon appear darker. White or pale colours are best for the salon.

MULTIPLE CHOICE QUESTIONS

1 A positive reactions to a predisposition test will indicate that a:
   (a) 'para' tint may be used
   (b) vegetable dye may not be used
   (c) nitro dye may be used
   (d) 'para' tint may not be used

2 Hydrogen peroxide is added to oxidation tints mainly to:
   (a) oxidize the natural pigment
   (b) open the cuticle scales
   (c) coat the hair shaft with colour
   (d) develop the colour of the tint

3 The top should be securely screwed back on to a tube of 'para' dye that has been opened to hinder:
   (a) hardening
   (b) oxidation
   (c) leakage
   (d) evaporation

4 After a normal regrowth application, tint is sometimes combed through to the ends to:
   (a) make the dye last longer
   (b) avoid the roots being too dark
   (c) restore lost or faded colour
   (d) prevent the colour fading

5 When applied to the hair, oxidation dyes:
   (a) add colour pigments to the cortex
   (b) remove colour pigments from the medulla
   (c) add colour pigments to the cuticle
   (d) coat the hair with coloured pigments

6 Colour reducers are used:
   (a) for pigmentation
   (b) to counteract the effect of artificial lighting
   (c) to remove oxidation tints from hair
   (d) as a reagent for the patch test

7 An oxidation dye may react with a client's skin to cause:
   (a) psoriasis
   (b) dermatitis (eczema)
   (c) ringworm
   (d) acid burns

8 Light produced by tungsten filament lamps contains more of which colour than does sunlight:
   (a) red
   (b) green
   (c) blue
   (d) yellow

9 Hair which has not been previously treated by hairdressing processes is known as:
   (a) acid balanced hair
   (b) normal hair
   (c) virgin hair
   (d) vellus hair

10 In order to dye the hair lighter than the natural colour, the strength of hydrogen peroxide added to the oxidation tint should be:
   (a) 10 vol. 3%
   (b) 20 vol. 6%
   (c) 30 vol. 9%
   (d) 40 vol. 12%

11 A red pigment will:
   (a) absorb green and reflect red
   (b) absorb red and reflect green
   (c) absorb magenta and reflect cyan
   (d) absorb heat and reflect the spectrum

12 Unwanted green or matt shades which develop during hair tinting may be corrected by adding a little:
   (a) blue
   (b) yellow
   (c) violet
   (d) red

13 An accelerator produces:
   (a) infra-red light
   (b) ultra-violet light
   (c) irradiated light
   (d) steam

14 When applying tint the hairdresser should wear protective gloves to prevent:
   (a) ringworm
   (b) contact dermatitis (eczema)
   (c) psoriasis
   (d) shingles

12
BLEACHING

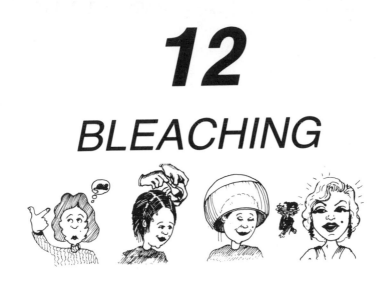

Hairdressers use bleach to lighten hair when other products (such as highlighting tints) are not strong enough. Remember, bleaching is a permanent process.

Clients who have naturally 'mousey' coloured hair which lightens in the sunlight, may often wish to re-achieve this effect. Blonde hair is often considered to be more flattering, especially with sun-tanned skin, and once clients have experienced blonde hair, they often feel that their own natural colour is less exciting.

Blonde highlights, especially on layered hair (where the natural colour regrowth is less obvious), are easier to sell to clients. The initial cost of highlights, especially woven highlights (which take more time) may be high, but they need be repeated only every few months. If clients prefer a full head bleach then the regrowth must be done every few weeks.

All bleaching processes are highly skilled, both in the analysis, mixing, application and development – so make sure you charge accordingly!

Bleaching chemical products will either partially or totally remove the natural pigments (melanin) in hair or can be used to lighten artificially coloured hair.

CHEMISTRY

Bleaches normally contain:

1   An **oxidizing agent** – usually hydrogen peroxide (H_2O_2). This breaks down to water and oxygen when it is slightly alkaline.

H_2O_2 alkaline $H_2O + O$
Hydrogen $\longrightarrow$ Water   Oxygen
peroxide

2   An **alkaline** – for example ammonium hydroxide, ammonium carbonate. This acts as a **catalyst** (a chemical which speeds up a chemical reaction and remains unchanged itself at the end of the reaction) to speed up the release of oxygen from hydrogen peroxide. The alkali is often thickened to form a paste bleach, an oil bleach or a cream bleach.

    The alkali and the oxidizing agent are mixed together immediately before use.

The effect of bleaching on the hair

The new oxygen released from the breakdown of hydrogen peroxide is a powerful bleaching agent. It combines chemically with the natural pigments in the hair to form coloured oxides. This is an **oxidation reaction**.

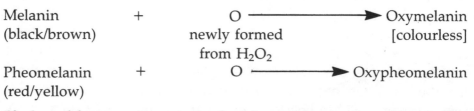

Melanin   +   O $\longrightarrow$ Oxymelanin
(black/brown)   newly formed   [colourless]
                    from H_2O_2
Pheomelanin   +   O $\longrightarrow$ Oxypheomelanin
(red/yellow)

Black and brown pigments (melanin) are more easily oxidized than red and yellow (pheomelanin) so that oxidation takes place in three stages:

black/brown $\longrightarrow$ red/yellow $\longrightarrow$ yellow

Hair, when bleached, will always lighten in this order:

black
dark brown
medium red brown
light warm brown
dark golden brown
medium golden blonde
light blonde
very light blonde
white – disintegration!

Hair must never be allowed to lighten beyond a very light blonde colour!

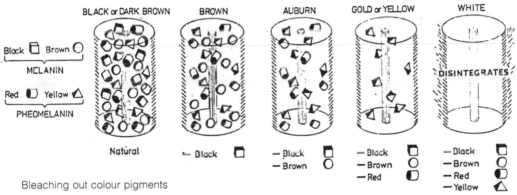

Bleaching out colour pigments

Unfortunately the hydrogen peroxide also oxidizes other parts of the internal structure of the hair. This can result in loss of strength and elasticity, hair breakage, increased porosity and roughened or destroyed cuticle scales. The aim of bleaching therefore is to öxidize the melanin with as little damage to the hair structure as possible.

After bleaching an antioxidant (reducing agent) rinse such as ascorbic acid is added. This has the added advantage of neutralizing any excess alkaline. Other conditioners or restructurants may also be used to help to repair damage to the hair.

ANALYSIS AND PREPARATION

Hair characteristics

Refer to the previous analysis chart (see page 203) regarding the hair texture, abundance, porosity, length, natural depth and tone of colour, the percentage and distribution of white hair, and any previous chemical treatments.

Although hair colouring is a controlled chemical process, in that the product will stop working after a period of time (e.g. 'para' dyes work for approximately 30 minutes), hair bleaches will continue to lighten hair for as long as they are in contact with the hair. It is possible tö lighten very dark hair to blonde in one application of strong bleach: but natural red pigments in the hair may prevent this from happening and two or three applications may be necessary.

Strand tests

These are taken in the same way as for hair colouring but bleach products are applied instead to test for the degree of lightness.

Sometimes it is necessary to test for tensile strength before bleaching by using a strand test (see page 204). Overbleached hair when wet is almost like chewing gum. When it is stretched (by pulling with your fingers) it will break off! Hair in this state will not be able to withstand any more bleaching.

Strand tests are also necessary to test for incompatibilities. This is when you suspect the client may have a hair colour restorer on her or his hair. The metallic salts from this product will produce steam and breakage if bleach is applied.

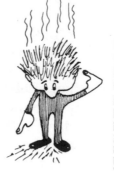

Sensitive scalps

Ask the client if she has a particularly sensitive scalp. If this is the case, then proceed with caution using lower peroxide strengths and milder bleach products where appropriate. Hydrogen peroxide will burn the skin and leave white patches which disappear with time, but most scalps can withstand this.

Examination of the scalp

Check the scalp for inflammation, cuts and abrasions and only continue if there are no contra-indications.

Discussion

First, discuss the style required by the client and then decide the appropriate method of bleaching, i.e. full head bleach, highlights, part-head bleach or for a fashion effect.

Generally older clients suit more subtle blonde tones such as light blonde, beige blonde and light golden beige or warm beige. Young clients often require white blonde or striking fashion colours such as pink, blue, green or purple (which are applied to bleached white hair).

Record cards

(See page 202.) Always check the client's previous records and ask every time if she was satisfied with the previous results. Clients' needs change with their lifestyles, e.g. job changes, new relationships, and even holiday needs (the sun will lighten bleached hair very quickly and dry it out), therefore different products and techniques may be needed.

New clients must be tactfully questioned about previous treatments – clients always remember bad experiences with their hair, especially bleaches, but rarely mention the good ones. If you suspect a client's hair to be particularly damaged always test first.

Gowning up

Gown up the client with a rubberized gown to prevent chemical splashes (these need frequent cleaning) and use towels, shoulder capes and tissues around the neck area. Remember that bleaches not only lighten hair but clothes too.

Clients with sensitive skins may also need protective 'barrier' cream applied around the hairline.

Remember to protect your own clothes with a dye apron and wear protective rubber gloves.

Work areas

Bleaches are normally applied at the dressing position, but may be mixed at the dispensary. Always prevent spillages by working cleanly and carefully. If any product is accidentally spilt on work surfaces (including the equipment trolley) or on the floor – wipe it up immediately. Remember bleaches can continue to be active for a long time and can cause skin burns.

EQUIPMENT

Bowls

See page 46.

Applicators

Bleaches may be applied with either tinting brushes (see page 46), applicator bottles with special nozzles or applicator guns. Check the manufacturer's instructions to see which to use. Always clean them thoroughly, rinse and dry after use.

Specialist tools

HIGHLIGHT CAP AND HOOK These special rubberized caps require frequent washing and powdering. Metal highlight hooks are available in various sizes according to the thickness of highlight required. Always keep the hooks in a noticeable place (e.g. a labelled container), as they are small and easily lost.

TIN FOIL Large rolls of tin foil are easily available, and must be cut to size and folded ready.

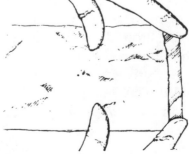

Special containers with rolls of foil available in the correct width are much quicker to prepare, as only the length need be cut ready. Never use hairdressing scissors to cut foil, it will ruin them! (See page 209.)

CLING PLASTIC Special heavy duty cling plastic is available to use for woven highlights, covering cap highlights or covering unbleached hair during part head bleaching. Cut the cling plastic to size beforehand.

SELF ADHESIVE PLASTIC STRIPS These useful strips stick to the hair underneath, bleach is then applied, then the packet is re-sealed. Choose the correct length of strip for the length of hair – long layered hair may need various sizes.

Foil, cling plastic and self-adhesive plastic strips are disposable and thrown away after use. (See page 209.)

Measures

See page 53.

Section clips

See page 47.

Cotton Wool

This is needed to clean away any bleach spilt onto either the client's hairline or protective cape. Remove the spilt product immediately.

Accelerator

See page 44. The accelerator speeds up the lightening process, but can dry the bleach products so that they become powdery if used for too long. Often plastic caps are used to cover the hair (especially over cap highlights to prevent the bleach from drying out).

Clients' scalps are often sensitized when bleach is applied – so take care when using an accelerator because of the risk of scalp burns.

Steamer

(See page 44.) Steamers are used to speed up the lightening process and because moist, moving air (steam) is emitted, it does not dry the bleach product and make it powdery. However, if the steamer is used for too long (more than 15–20 minutes), the steam will start to dilute the product, making it very runny.

MATERIALS

Use all bleach products strictly in accordance with the manufacturer's instructions.

Different bleach products will give varying degrees of lifting power (see Depth and Tone Chart, page 206). The natural colour depth is very important, i.e. to lift one shade means to lift, for example from Depth 8 to Depth 7, and to lift 3–4 shades means to lift, for example, from Depth 5 to Depth 7 or 8.

Remember when using hydrogen peroxide (mixed with bleach or colour products) – 20 Vol./6% or 30 Vol./9% is considered safe to touch the scalp, but 40 Vol./12% and higher volumes of peroxide are not considered safe to touch the scalp, but can be used carefully for highlights, or other methods not having scalp contact.

Oil bleach

This is a gentle bleach which will lift the hair 3–4 shades, and is mixed with either 20 vol./6% or 30 Vol./9% hydrogen peroxide. Oil bleaches are often mixed with shampoos and applied to towel dried hair to generally brighten it up. This brightening shampoo is only left on the hair for a short time.

Emulsion/gel/cream bleaches

These are stronger bleaches which will lift 5–6 shades and are mixed with either 20 Vol./6% or 30 Vol./9% hydrogen peroxide.

Sometimes special boosters or activators (containing sodium and ammonium persulphate) are mixed with emulsion or gel bleaches to give the bleach extra strength. Always check the manufacturer's instructions to see how many boosters or activators should be mixed for the amount of lift needed. Always check the order of mixing, for instance the hydrogen peroxide and the boosters or activators may need to be mixed before the emulsion or gel bleach is added – thus preventing a lumpy mixture which is difficult to apply.

Emulsion or gel bleaches are particularly good for whole head, regrowth and part head bleaches because of their consistency.

Powder bleaches (paste bleach)

These are strong bleaches (made from magnesium and sodium carbonate powders) which will lift from 6–8 shades, and are mixed with either 20 Vol./6%, 30 Vol./9% or 40 Vol./12% hydrogen peroxide.

They are often used for highlights and fashion effects, but do have a tendency to dry out and become powdery if excessive heat is applied.

Both powder and emulsion/gel bleaches are often blue in colour (although some manufacturers make a white powder). The problem with using blue coloured bleaches is that silver/blue neutralizes yellow/orange which is the colour of the bleached hair (see page 212). Therefore it is often very difficult to see the correct degree of lightness without removing the bleach product from the hair.

Oxidizers

Hydrogen peroxide is the most common oxidizer used when bleaching. It is available in both liquid and cream liquid form. Sometimes it is necessary to dilute liquid peroxide from a stronger to a weaker solution if the correct strength is unavailable.

Make sure you use the correct strength of hydrogen peroxide according to the manufacturer's instructions.

STORAGE OF HYDROGEN PEROXIDE Hydrogen peroxide decomposes to water and oxygen very easily. Light, heat and exposure to air will all speed up its decomposition. Because of this, manufacturers add acid to the hydrogen peroxide for salon use. This acid acts as a **stabilizer** to prevent premature breakdown.

However, correct storage conditions for hydrogen peroxide are still vital to ensure that it retains its strength.

1   Store in cool, dry conditions.
2   Store in opaque (no light can get through) or dark containers.

3   Replace stopper tightly immediately after use.
4   Always store away from inflammable materials. The oxygen given off by decomposing hydrogen peroxide can assist fires.

STRENGTH OF HYDROGEN PEROXIDE The strength of hydrogen peroxide solution may be measured as percentage strength (%) or volume strength (vol.).

The higher the volume strength (vol.) or percentage strength (%) of hydrogen peroxide (H_2O_2) the more oxygen is given off, e.g. 1 litre of 10 vol. (3%) H_2O_2 will give off 10 litres of oxygen and leave 1 litre of water $H_2O_2 \rightarrow H_2O+O$.

Since it is this oxygen which is given off from the hydrogen peroxide that brings about the oxidation process, the higher the concentration of hydrogen peroxide, the stronger the result.

10 vol. = 3%   20 vol. = 6%   30 vol. = 9%

40 vol. = 12%   60 vol. = 18%

A **peroxometer** (a type of hydrometer) may be used to test the strength of the hydrogen peroxide (perhaps it is old stock or has not been stored properly). Peroxometers only work with liquid hydrogen peroxide, not liquid cream.

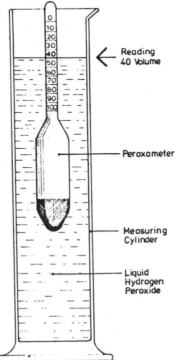

DILUTION OF HYDROGEN PEROXIDE   If the correct strength of hydrogen peroxide is not available it may be necessary to dilute a higher strength of hydrogen peroxide to that required. Ideally distilled water should be used for dilution.

The following examples show an easy way to do dilutions:

1   To obtain 30 vol. hydrogen peroxide from a solution in stock of 60 vol:
    Take 30 ml of stock H_2O_2 and make it up to 60 ml (i.e. add a further 30 ml of water.)

2   To obtain 20 vol. hydrogen peroxide from a solution in stock of 60 vol:
    Take 20 ml of stock H_2O_2 and make it up to 60 ml (i.e. add a further 40 ml of water).

3   To obtain 30 vol. hydrogen peroxide from a solution in stock of 40 vol:
    Take 30 ml of stock H_2O_2 and make it up to 40 ml (i.e. add a further 10 ml of water).

4   To obtain 10 vol. hydrogen peroxide from a solution in stock of 40 vol:
    Take 10 ml of stock H_2O_2 and make it up to 40 ml (i.e. add a further 30 ml of water).

Stock solution	Required solution	Quantity of stock solution	Quantity + of water	Total final quantity and volume strength
100 vol.	→ 60 vol.	60 ml	+40 ml	100 ml of 60 vol.
100 vol.	→ 40 vol.	40 ml	+60 ml	100 ml of 40 vol.
100 vol.	→ 30 vol.	30 ml	+70 ml	100 ml of 30 vol.
100 vol.	→ 20 vol.	20 ml	+80 ml	100 ml of 20 vol.
60 vol.	→ 40 vol.	40 ml	+20 ml	60 ml of 40 vol.
40 vol.	→ 30 vol.	30 ml	+10 ml	40 ml of 30 vol.
40 vol.	› 20 vol.	20 ml	+20 ml	40 ml of 20 vol.
30 vol.	→ 20 vol.	20 ml	+10 ml	30 ml of 20 vol.

Any quantity can be used instead of mls, e.g. pints, fluid ounces, centilitres, etc. Dilutions involving percentage strengths instead of volume strengths are calculated in the same way.

Occasionally, oxidizers may be obtained in the form of small crystals, but these are mild oxidizers and are used for mixing with bleach toners (see page 236).

METHODS AND TECHNIQUES

Whole head bleaching

Both whole head and regrowth bleaches are usually applied to hair
sectioned into four.

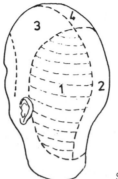

Sections for bleaching

Bleach is usually applied to the nape area first where the hair is more
resistent. For a whole head application of bleach to virgin hair the
technique is the same as that for tinting, i.e. apply to: the mid-lengths,
the points or the ends, the roots.

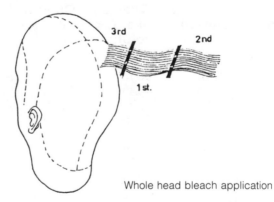

Whole head bleach application

This is because the client's body heat (from her scalp) will enable the
product applied there to take more quickly.

Never skimp with the amount of bleach used and take smaller
sections than when tinting — the smallest area left uncovered with
the product will show up disastrously! Always check the application
thoroughly.

Regrowth application

Some manufacturers will stipulate that the product should be applied with a bowl and brush, whilst others state than an applicator bottle with a nozzle should be used.

Whilst applying to a regrowth, which must always be thorough, never overlap onto the previously bleached hair, as hair breakage could occur.

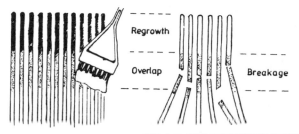

Clients with large regrowths (over 20 mm long) may need two applications of bleach to prevent 'banding'   uneven colour result. First apply the bleach to the dark hair (15 mm away from the roots) thoroughly, then apply the bleach to the root area. This is because the client's body heat would make the root area take too quickly.

Part head bleaching

To achieve a fashion effect only part of the head is bleached. Use the same technique as for whole head bleaching (i.e. mid-lengths, points, then roots), but separating and covering the unbleached hair by the same method as block-colouring.

Checking the application

You can never be too careful when applying bleach, always check the application in the opposite direction from the way in which you applied it.

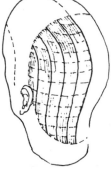

If you have missed any areas, apply bleach to them immediately — or dark patches will be seen. Pay special attention to the hairline and the thickest parts of the hair (i.e. behind the ears).

Checking the client's skin

If any bleach has accidentally come into contact with the client's face, ears or neck — remove it immediately. Bleach products entering the client's eyes must be removed immediately by running water or an eye wash (see page 9).

Client comfort

Bleaching can be a long, drawn-out process, so make sure your client is warm and comfortable and offer refreshments and magazines during the development time.

Development

TIMING Time the development according to the manufacturer's directions. Remember that both warm and cold salon conditions and over-porous hair can affect the timing — so do not leave the client unattended. Ask the client if her scalp is comfortable (especially when applying bleach to the scalp area) and check the hair lightening development.

It is difficult to test the degree of lightness required during bleaching as some bleaches are blue in colour (see page 227) and poor salon lighting (see page 214) can affect your judgement.

Always remove some of the bleach product from a strand of hair with damp cotton wool and water. Wipe dry with cotton wool, then lay the strand of hair over a fresh piece of dry cotton wool. This is the best way to see the true degree of lightness obtained. If the hair is not light enough then re-apply the bleach and continue to develop it.

Hairdressers often do a tensile strength test at this stage, using their fingers, to test the amount of elasticity in the hair.

USE OF STEAMER/ACCELERATOR See page 44. Steamers and accelerators give extra heat, and generally cut the development time by half. To prevent some products from drying out a disposable plastic bag may be used to cover the hair during highlighting.

Fashion techniques

Once you are successful and confident with bleaching, there are many varied techniques to choose from. Always style the hair first, then decide where the lightened areas will look most effective.

SLICING   This technique involves taking slices of hair, wrapping them in foil or self-adhesive strips and applying the bleach — without seepage. To prevent seepage wrap the packets around the root area with either extra strips of foil or thin strips of cotton wool. This is because bleach is permanent and difficult to rectify if any seepage does occur.

The sections for slicing will depend on the style chosen. Always work methodically using either section clips or butterfly clips to hold the hair.

When the product is developed, remove by shampooing. Colour products (coppers, reds, pinks, blues, greens, yellows) may be applied at this stage if a more vibrant look is required.

SCRUNCHING   This is a fun technique used to produce lightened ends very quickly. It works best on curly, layered hair which has been dressed into style.

The bleach must be of a thick consistency and is applied with your fingertips; sectioning is not necessary. Protective gloves must be worn and the bleach is dappled over the ends of the hair, developed and shampooed out. Colour products may again be applied at this stage (see Slicing).

All fashion techniques must be applied with care as bleach products expand during development (due to the oxygen being liberated) and seepage can easily occur and ruin the look.

Highlighting

Highlights also have the advantage that no product touches the scalp, which is useful for clients with sensitive scalps.

THE CAP METHOD   Always brush the hair into the finished style before putting the cap on. This will ensure that the highlights show in the correct areas of hair.

Check that the highlights cap is suitable for your use. If the client requires thick highlights (thick, abundant hair may need them to be heavy to show up), then a previously used cap will be better. However, many clients prefer fine highlights (which look good on fine hair) and a new highlight cap with less enlarged holes is more suitable. If the cap has torn or enlarged holes — disregard it. Remember the problems of bleach seepage!

Sometimes it is painful for the client when a highlight cap is put on, as it must be fixed securely and as close to the scalp as possible. A little talcum powder sprinkled on to the cap, or a little dressing cream or conditioner applied to the hair, will make the cap easier to put on.

Strands of hair are then pulled through the cap with a highlight hook. Start pulling the strands through from the edges of the cap to check the required thickness. This way, if the strands are too thick, they can easily be pulled back under the cap again with the highlight hook.

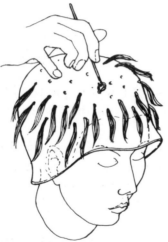

Once all the strands have been pulled through — mix the bleach. If done before the product would have oxidized prematurely and not be strong enough.

The bleach is then applied thoroughly to all the hair strands, checked, then developed.

WOVEN HIGHLIGHTS   This skilled technique takes time, but is more precise than the cap method in that the hairdresser can see exactly where the highlights are being placed. The product can also be applied closer to the root area than with the cap method. This is why most salons charge more for woven highlights.

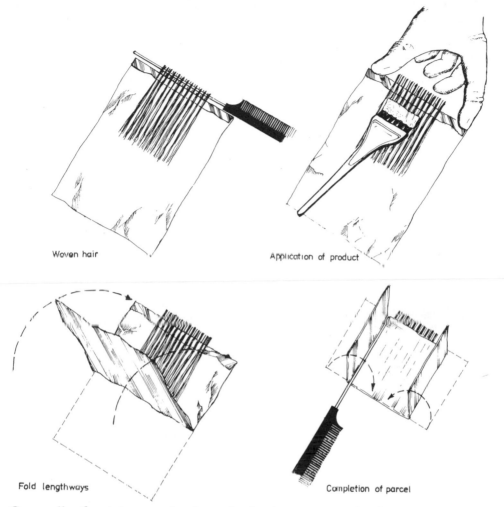

Woven hair   Application of product

Fold lengthways   Completion of parcel

Generally the 'nine section' method of preparing the hair (see page 177) is used so that you can work methodically.

Either foil or self adhesive strips are used to hold the hair which is woven out with a pin-tail comb.

Always check when weaving out the strands of hair that the strand directly below is not woven, or else the client will end up with stripes! This is quite difficult to achieve as a sub-section of hair is always left out between each woven section. The sub-sections for weaving out highlights are similar depths to those used for perming (i.e. the size of a small perm rod).

As this is a lengthy process, some of the highlights may have developed to the required degree of lightness before completion, so check the development continually (see page 231). If some highlights are ready, then stop the development on those strands only. This is done by removing the product with cotton wool and warm water, then continue weaving the other highlights and applying the product. Sometimes, re-mixing bleach is necessary as it will lose its strength after a time. Develop and remove the bleach as normal.

TIPPING   This is a similar technique to woven highlights, but the small meshes of hair are wrapped individually in foil parcels. Either the whole length or the ends of the mesh can be bleached to achieve various effects.

Tipped streaks are generally thicker and more obvious than woven or cap highlights.

Removing the bleach

SHAMPOOING   Remove the bleach product by rinsing thoroughly until the water runs clear. Use a lower water temperature than usual because the client's scalp will be sensitive, but ask the client if the temperature is comfortable. Give one or two shampoos, according to the manufacturer's instructions.

Bleach toners

If the client requires a bleach toner then do not condition the hair. Towel dry the hair after shampooing, disentangle it and remove the client from the washbasin to the dressing position.

Choose the colour toner with your client (see Colouring Analysis, page 203) but take into account the degree of lightness required.

Generally, a pale yellow depth needs either ash, soft grey, or beige tones, whereas a very pale yellow depth needs a mauve, blue or silver tone.

If you are applying the bleach toner to cap highlights do not remove the highlight cap.

Remember the hair is very porous at this stage and generally weak. Volumes of hydrogen peroxide (10 vol./3% or 20 vol./6%) are mixed with bleach toners. They are often applied with special applicator bottles so that they are applied quickly as they can develop sooner than expected. Never leave a bleach toner during the development time — once it has 'grabbed' an over porous hair, it is very difficult to remove (see colour reduction, page 213).

Fashion colours

(See Slicing, page 233 for pinks, blues, greens and yellows.) Coppers and reds are often applied to pre-bleached hair to achieve a more vibrant affect.

The hair need only be pre-bleached to an orange/yellow depth to apply warm copper tones, and pre-bleached to an orange/red depth to apply auburn, bright copper or clear red tones.

Always follow the manufacturer's directions very closely for fashion colours: they include direct stain dyes and are not mixed with hydrogen peroxide (see page 245).

The method of application is the same as for bleach toners (but check if the hair has to be towel dried, or dry beforehand).

Conditioning

An anti-oxy acid rinse (such as ascorbic acid) may be used to stop all bleaching activity. However, bleaching always leaves the hair more porous and it often needs extra conditioning after shampooing. Remember the client's comfort. A sensitive scalp will be sore if the hair has to be disentangled without any conditioner.

Gently squeeze any excess water from the hair, and apply either a conditioner or a restructurant.

Record card

The client's record card is completed at this stage and filed for future use.

UNDESIRABLE EFFECTS FOLLOWING BLEACHING

Bleaching fault	Cause
Hair damage/breakage	1 Applying bleach (overlapping) onto previously bleached hair (see page 231). 2 Incorrect mixing, proportions of mixture incorrect or too many boosters/activators used (see page 226). 3 Too high volumes of hydrogen peroxide used (see page 228). 4 Over-developing the bleach — leaving it on too long (see page 232). 5 Not taking a strand test (see page 222).
Skin/scalp damage	1 Not using barrier cream around the client's hairline (see page 180). 2 Incorrect mixing, proportions of mixture incorrect or too many boosters/activators used (see page 226). 3 Too high volumes of hydrogen peroxide used (see page 228). 4 Over-developing the bleach — leaving it on too long (see page 232).
Hair not light enough	1 Incorrect analysis of natural hair colour — depth and tone (see page 206) 2 Incorrect choice of bleach product to lighten (see page 226). 3 Bleach mixed too soon before application (see page 226) 4 Insufficient development time (see page 232).
Hair overlightened	1 Incorrect analysis of natural hair colour — depth and tone (see page 206). 2 Incorrect choice of bleach product to lighten (see page 226).
Uneven colour result: From bleach product	1 Insufficient product used (see page 236). 2 Application not checked thoroughly (see page 231). 3 Large regrowth bleach applied incorrectly (see page 231).
From bleach toner, or fashion colour	1 Incorrect hair preparation (see page 236–7). 2 Incorrect mixing of product (see page 227). 3 Incorrect application of product (see page 236–7). 4 Incorrect timing of product (see page 236–7).

MULTIPLE CHOICE QUESTIONS

1 A chemical which speeds up chemical reactions and remains unchanged itself at the end of the reaction is called:
   (a)   an oxidizing agent
   (b)   a hydrolysing agent
   (c)   an alkali
   (d)   a catalyst

2 The effect of hydrogen peroxide on melanin is to:
   (a)   convert it to oxymelanin
   (b)   wash it away
   (c)   convert it to pheomelanin
   (d)   reduce it

3 Chemically speaking, the bleaching process is:
   (a)   a hydrolizing reaction
   (b)   a neutralization
   (c)   an oxidation reaction
   (d)   a reduction reaction

4 A reducing agent such as ascorbic acid is added after bleaching to:
   (a)   open the cuticle scales
   (b)   stop the reaction of hydrogen peroxide
   (c)   repair damage to the cortex
   (d)   cool the hair down

5 Hydrogen peroxide breaks down into:
   (a)   hydrogen and oxygen
   (b)   hydrogen and water
   (c)   oxygen and persulphate
   (d)   oxygen and water

6 Stabilizers added to prevent premature breakdown of hydrogen peroxide are:
   (a)   acid
   (b)   alkaline
   (c)   gels
   (d)   boosters

7 20 vol. hydrogen peroxide is equal to which % strength?
   (a)   3%
   (b)   6%
   (c)   9%
   (d)   12%

8 To say that a solution of hydrogen peroxide is 30 vol. means:
   (a)   that 1 ml of hydrogen peroxide liberates 30 ml oxygen
   (b)   30 mls of the solution should be used
   (c)   the solution is equal to a 30% solution
   (d)   30 mls of hydrogen peroxide liberate 1 ml of oxygen

9 To obtain 10 vol. hydrogen peroxide from 60 vol. take:
   (a)   10 ml (60 vol.) hydrogen peroxide and add 100 ml water
   (b)   50 ml (60 vol.) hydrogen peroxide and add 10 ml water
   (c)   10 ml (60 vol.) hydrogen peroxide and add 50 ml water
   (d)   1 ml hydrogen peroxide and add 600 ml water

10 Overlapping can cause:
   (a)   hair breakage
   (b)   traction alopecia
   (c)   folliculitis
   (d)   dermatitis

11 For cap highlights when should the bleach be mixed:
   (a)   before all the strands have been pulled through
   (b)   after all the strands have been pulled through
   (c)   before putting on the cap
   (d)   when half the strands have been pulled through

12 When bleaching the head, sectioning is necessary to ensure:
   (a)   correct processing time
   (b)   oxidation does not occur too rapidly
   (c)   a methodical procedure
   (d)   the correct amount of lightening

13 The highest concentration (volume) of hydrogen peroxide that should be allowed to touch the scalp is:
   (a)   10 vol. (3%)
   (b)   20 vol. (6%)
   (c)   30 vol. (9%)
   (d)   60 vol. (18%)

14 Barrier cream should be used around the client's hairline to prevent:
   (a)   damage to the eyes
   (b)   lightening of the skin colour
   (c)   damage to the hair
   (d)   damage to the skin

13

NON-PERMANENT COLOURING

In the salon these colours are known as temporary and semi-permanent hair colours. They are very exciting to use and create instant hair colour changes. However, the inexperienced hairdresser occasionally finds that they can become either permanent or very patchy.

TEMPORARY COLOURS

Types of synthetic dyes

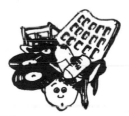

These may take a variety of forms.

Gels/Foams	Setting lotions, etc.	Water rinses	Coloured hairsprays
Dyes; coloured mousses and gels.	Coloured plastic setting lotions and blow dry lotions.	Concentrated colour drops and very hot water.	These may include gold and silver which contain metallic particles.

Synthetic dyes are good for introducing clients to hair colours, as they are quick to apply and easy to remove if the client is dissatisfied with the change. These may contain Azo dyes which give red-brown tones and basic dyes which give blue-violet tones.

Natural vegetable dyes

There are two main vegetable dyes used — Camomile and Henna.

CAMOMILE Camomile gives yellow/gold tones. It is a daisy-like plant which grows wild in the country. The flowers contain the golden-yellow dye, Apigenin. This is rarely used as a natural product but is often added to other products, e.g. shampoos and conditioners.

HENNA (see Chapter 11) One small application of henna, for example in a colour shampoo, may be considered to be a temporary or semi-permanent colour to give auburn highlights to brown hair. Remember repeated applications (especially on over-porous hair) make it a permanent colour.

Chemistry

The molecules of temporary dyes are too large to penetrate the cuticle and enter the hair shaft, so they coat the outside of the hair. This is why they are washed away so easily (see diagram, page 243).

Uses of temporary dyes

Temporary dyes are useful for adding stronger tones, e.g. warm, golden, ashen or silver tones to natural or artificially coloured hair.

Sometimes natural white hair or bleached hair looks too yellow or golden (brassy) and will benefit from the silver tones (see Colour Cancellation, page 212). However, for clients who wish to blend in a few stray grey hairs (remember grey hair is white and naturally coloured hair mixed together) it may be more difficult. Some colours produce unwanted warm (orange/red) overtones on the white hair — so take a strand test if in doubt (see page 204). They may also be used to darken naturally and artificially coloured hair.

Fashion colours and effects can be achieved very successfully using the techniques of block colouration (part-head colours) or woven highlights (see page 234), or even cap highlights (see page 233).

After discussion with the client, choose the appropriate non-permanent colour for the client explaining the benefits of each — remember the cost involved. As these products are quick and easy to apply, they are easy to sell.

SEMI-PERMANENT COLOURS

There are two types of semi-permanent colours:

foaming — applied from the container or with a sponge;
and liquid cream — applied using a bowl and brush.

These colours clean, colour and condition the hair at the same time and are useful for giving colour tone. Products often contain a detergent and conditioner as well as dye molecules.

They are non-allergic — a skin test is not needed, and they do not interfere with other hairdressing processes. Remember no peroxide is added to them. They last longer than temporary colourants, usually six to eight shampoos and they leave no regrowth. They will only cover 10-20% of the white hair present.

Chemistry

Semi-permanent colourants consist of small molecule dyes which are able to penetrate inside the cortex. They are not very soluble in water and so they tend to wash out slowly. They consist of mixtures of nitro dyes (red and yellow colours) and anthraquinones (blue colours).

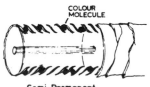

Semi-Permanent

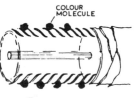

Temporary

Temporary and semi-permanent colour molecules

Discussion

Try to interest the client in non-permanent colourings either by using them yourself, or by displaying show cards, shade charts or style books.

Always take into consideration the client's skin tone or colour (see page 205).

Clients often have a preference for certain hair colours — sometimes it may be to suit a special occasion (e.g. a dinner dance) whilst other times it may be to match their outfit!

ANALYSIS

See Hair Colour Analysis, page 203. Although record cards are always kept to record colour details, these may not be available for new clients. Therefore, you need to question the client thoroughly, especially if you suspect that she may have coloured her hair at home. Look at the natural hair colour at the roots — if it is a different from the ends, then it is possible that she has had colour applied.

In the same way that the client's natural colour depth and tone are analyzed for permanent colours, manufacturers produce colour charts to guide both you and the client towards a decision. Some colour charts (or shade guides) even have samples of the client's natural colour and the completed colour on that sample. This is very important as, for instance, a light silver blonde looks good on light blonde hair but would not even show up on dark brown hair. Likewise, a copper tone may appear suitable for light brown hair, but would be far too bright on white hair.

Examination of hair and scalp

Check the scalp for cuts, abrasions, inflammation, infections or infestations.

Some non-permanent colours may tend to stain the scalp. If the client's scalp is excessively dry, rectify that problem before applying the colour (see page 163).

Check the hair for porosity (over-porous and non-porous), texture, length, abundance (see page 204), and decide the natural depth and tone of colour (see page 206). If the hair is artificially coloured then look at that and any natural colour appearing at the regrowth area. Always assess the amount of white hair present.

Strand tests

(See page 204.) Incompatibility test cuttings are unnecessary for non-permanent colours because they are not mixed with hydrogen peroxide.

However, to give the clients confidence and to reassure yourself, it may be useful to take a strand test to see the final colour. This is done in the same way as described in Chapter 11, but the appropriate non-permanent colour is applied instead.

Gowning up

Always protect the client with appropriate gowns, towels and shoulder capes, as some non-permanent colours can be very runny and difficult to use. Make sure that your clothes are properly protected with a dye apron, non-permanent colours are sometimes called **stain dyes.** Likewise, you must wear protective gloves to prevent both your nails and hands from becoming stained.

Barrier cream may be applied to the client's hairline as a protection against skin straining, but take care not to apply any to the client's hair or the colour will not penetrate and 'take'.

Work areas

Sometimes these colours are applied at the washbasin, whilst at other times the dressing position may be used. Wipe up any product that may have split onto the surrounding working areas and floors immediately. In the same way that these colours can stain your hands, they can stain all surfaces — that includes the client's clothes and skin too!

EQUIPMENT

If the colour is applied at the dressing position, then the equipment trolley will be needed. Place all the necessary equipment in the trays below in case of spillage and use the top tray.

If the manufacturer specifies that a bowl and brush or bowl and sponge are to be used make sure that they are always clean and dry before and after use.

Sectioning clips may be needed to section the hair if necessary, and cotton wool is useful for cleansing around the front and back hairline to remove skin stains.

Some manufacturers state that plastic caps (see page 46) may be necessary during processing to control any body heat. Accelerators and steamers (see page 44) are sometimes used to speed up the colouring process.

METHOD FOR TEMPORARY COLOURS

Application

The gels/foams, setting lotions and water rinses are applied according to the manufacturer's directions. Shampoo first, then towel dry the hair. For complete control of the colour apply using a bowl and brush.

Coloured hair sprays, gels and paints are applied during dressing and are used for special occasions.

Removal

Removal is by shampooing out. The colour is washed out at the first shampoo.

METHOD FOR SEMI-PERMANENT COLOURS

For semi-permanent colours you should give one or two soapless shampoos and towel dry the hair, or the application may be uneven, as excess water dilutes the product.

Amount of product

Some products are applied directly from an applicator bottle, and may be supplied in individual containers. If too little product is supplied (for instance the client may have long hair and need two bottles to be used), then do not skimp with the product — use extra and charge accordingly. If the product is only available in large containers — use the appropriate amount but do not waste products.

Sectioning

Divide the hair into fairly large sub-sections if specified by the manufacturer. Secure the sub-sections with either section clips or butterfly clips.

Mixing

Mix an appropriate amount of colour according to the technique selected.

Sub-sectioning

Take neat, even partings, meshes or sections as appropriate. Generally abundant hair and products with a thick consistency need smaller sub-sections, and vice-versa.

Checking the application

Cross check the application (see page 231) to see that all the hair has been covered with the product.

Ensure that the colour has not come into contact with any other areas, i.e. the face, neck, ears or eyes.

Development

Always make sure that the hair is sufficiently loosened to allow the circulation of air or to allow warmth from either an accelerator or a steamer to penetrate.

Always check the hair colour development by removing some product from a few strands of hair with damp cotton wool and placing the hair over a clean piece of cotton wool. Remember over-porous hair develops quickly.

The development time will vary from manufacturer to manufacturer — so check the instructions. Most semi-permanent colours are left from 2-20 minutes to develop.

Removal

Most semi-permanent colours are removed by thorough rinsing with warm water as the hair has already been shampooed — but always check the manufacturer's instructions and feel the hair to make sure it is clean.

Generally, conditioning agents are added to semi-permanent colours, but if the hair is tangled or matted, use either a conditioner or a restructurant (see page 161).

Complete the record card at this stage.

UNDESIRABLE EFFECTS FOLLOWING NON-PERMANENT HAIR COLOURING

Undesirable effects can be avoided. Check the following points:

Colour fault	Cause
Incorrect colour result	1 Incorrect understanding of manufacturer's instructions regarding choice of colour according to client's natural colour (i.e. depth of tone and percentage of white hair present). 2 Failure to show the client the manufacturer's shade chart whilst discussing the target colour. 3 Incorrect analysis of hair (see page 244).
Skin staining	1 Colour used on an excessively dry scalp. 2 Barrier cream not used around the client's hairline.
Insufficient hair coverage/patchy result	1 Incorrect choice of product (generally foam colours are easier and quicker to apply to over-porous hair). 2 Incorrect choice of colour — no strand test taken 3 Insufficient timing during development or product left on far too long without checking. 4 Incorrect application — check the manufacturer's instructions — i.e. semi-permanents that foam up should be applied with a bowl and sponge not a bowl and brush.

Corrective techniques

Sometimes, especially if the hair is very porous, some of the dye molecules may be taken up or remain within the hair shaft even though the other dye molecules have been washed away. This may give rise to colour distortions or patchy results. If the non-permanent colour has 'grabbed' in this way on the hair then try:

1   Repeated shampooing.
2   Using white spirit and cotton wool (to dry hair).
3   A brightening shampoo (10 vol./3% hydrogen peroxide and shampoo in equal parts).

MULTIPLE CHOICE QUESTIONS

1 Which of the following is likely to give an uneven result when a direct dye is applied:
  (a)   fine hair
  (b)   dry hair
  (c)   coarse hair
  (d)   bleached hair
2 A temporary dye of vegetable origin is:
  (a)   camomile
  (b)   Henna
  (c)   azo dye
  (d)   calamine
3 In which part of the hair are temporary dyes normally deposited?
  (a)   cortex
  (b)   medulla
  (c)   cuticle
  (d)   dermal papilla
4 Coloured setting lotions usually contain:
  (a)   'para' dyes
  (b)   azo dyes
  (c)   metallic dyes
  (d)   vegetable dyes

5 Nitro dyes and anthraquinones are examples of:
  (a) temporary acidic dyes
  (b) temporary basic dyes
  (c) mineral dyes
  (d) semi-permanent dyes
6 The active ingredient in henna is:
  (a) lawsone
  (b) hydrogen peroxide
  (c) ammonium hydroxide
  (d) lanette wax
7 Pale pastel dyes applied to highly bleached hair are often quickly lost because the:
  (a) hydrogen peroxide cannot close the cuticle
  (b) hair is too porous to hold them
  (c) natural pigments have been removed
  (d) hair has been weakened by bleaching
8 Semi-permanent dyes easily penetrate into the hair fibre because they:
  (a) have small molecules
  (b) have electrostatic charges
  (c) dissolve in water
  (d) are attracted to keratin

14

DESIGN PRINCIPLES

An understanding of art is not necessary to be able to design hairstyles. However, without a knowledge of the principles of design related to hairstyles, face-shapes, body proportions and salon interiors, you cannot be a good practising hairdresser.

Line, volume, shape and proportion, texture and colour are all part of the planning necessary to achieve a hairstyle which suits the client.

Fashions change very quickly, and hairdressers who have been practising for some years have to be able to adapt constantly. Therefore, a historical knowledge of hairstyles is very useful; not only the method used to achieve the style, but an understanding of the 'total look'. Certain styles suit some outfits better than others, for example, an Edwardian wedding dress looks better with an upswept or curled hairstyle rather than a square bob.

DESIGNING A HAIRSTYLE

Lines

Lines can be straight, curled, angular, blurred, thick, thin and parallel. During sectioning for styling, cutting, perming, colouring and bleaching, thick and thin paralled lines are often made through the hair.

Partings in a style can alter the client's image.

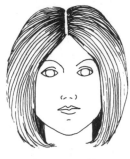

A centre parting
lengthens the face

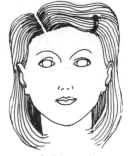

A side parting
broadens the face

FRONT LINES

Horizontal   These lines are good for straight hair with no unusual hair growth patterns (see Chapter 8).

Curved   Curved lines are usually cut just above the eyebrows and help to slim down wide foreheads.

Angular   'V' shaped lines, where the hair flicks back off the face are often flattering, since it creates fullness and lift.

Blurred   When the hair is taken back from the front hairline, the line is often uneven and blurred. It is most suitable for short hair, but can be used for long haired dressings. It will highlight all the client's features.

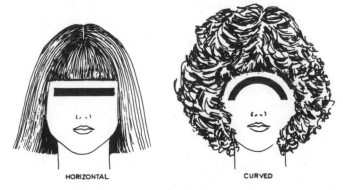

HORIZONTAL   CURVED

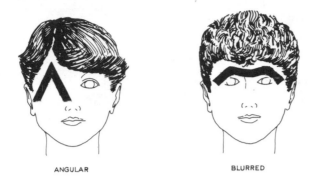

ANGULAR   BLURRED

SIDELINES

Horizontal   Square lines cut horizontally through the hair can be cut all one length or half way through the hairstyle.

One length horizontal lines will hide both cheekbones and jawlines, whereas hair cut away towards the ears will make them more noticeable.

Diagonal   Diagonal lines away from the face expose the cheeks and jawline, but are more flattering than horizontal lines. Diagonal lines dropping towards the face throw hair weight towards the face and create an illusion of lengthening the neck while hiding the profile.

Curved   Curved shapes are produced either from hair being cut very short against the hairline or being styled back away from the hairline, exposing all the features.

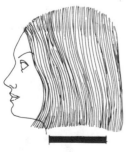

HORIZONTAL

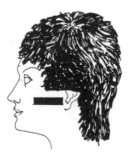

HORIZONTAL

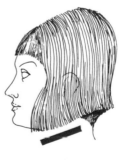

DIAGONAL

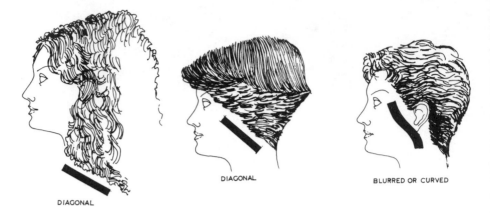

DIAGONAL

DIAGONAL

BLURRED OR CURVED

BACK LINES

Horizontal These lines often cover the back hairline and are useful for longer hair, giving lift to the profile.

Angular A 'V' shaped line is very practical as shorter sides and longer hair at the back are very easy for clients to manage at home. It will also give the illusion of narrowing down a wide neck and shoulders.

Curved Convex shapes are useful to give a practical style which does not catch on a client's collar, while still appearing long from the front view.

Blurred Short, soft hairlines are very practical and easy for the client to manage. However, natural hair growth patterns (see Chapter 8) will always dictate the direction in which the hair will lie.

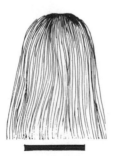

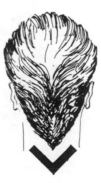

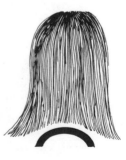

HORIZONTAL

ANGULAR

CURVED

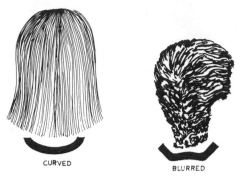

CURVED   BLURRED

Volume

Volume can be created within a hairstyle through backcombing or backbrushing (see page 120), or by club or taper cutting the hair (see page 135).

Larger volumes of hair can be achieved by using postiche (wigs or hairpieces) or by supporting the hair with frames made of wire or card.

Shape

The shape of a hairstyle can be rounded, geometric, jagged or smooth.

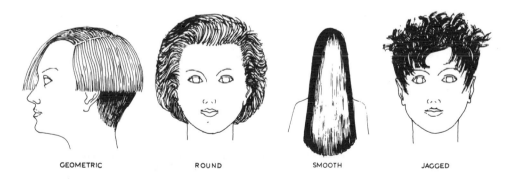

GEOMETRIC   ROUND   SMOOTH   JAGGED

Proportion/balance

To achieve a good proportion in a hairstyle it must be balanced i.e. one part of it must balance against another part, and the hairstyle must balance the face and body proportions.

Fashion styles may be symmetric, i.e. level or asymmetric, i.e. unlevel.

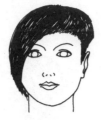

An asymmetric style

Texture

The texture of hair can be felt (either coarse or soft) or seen to be either smooth or fluffy. Straight hair often appears smooth and shiny, whereas wavy or curly hair often looks fluffy and dull.

Hair may be smoothed or curled during styling by setting, blow styling or by using heated styling equipment.

Styling aids such as gel, mousse, dressing creams and hairspray will also change the appearance of the texture of the hair.

Colour

(See Chapters 11, 12 and 13.)

There are **primary colours**, i.e. red, yellow and blue and **secondary colours**, i.e. orange (red and yellow) green (yellow and blue) mauve (red and blue).

For hair colouring we say that colour pigments are either warm (containing red), cold (do not contain red) or neutral (i.e. light to dark base shades 1–10 on the ICC shade chart) (see page 206).

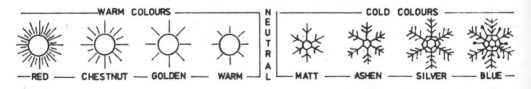

Complementary colours are those which cancel each other out to produce a neutral colour (see page 212).

Harmonious colours are those close together on the colour circle, e.g. red and red-violet.

Colour tones mean how light or how dark each tone is, this can be achieved graphically by using the 'dot' technique.

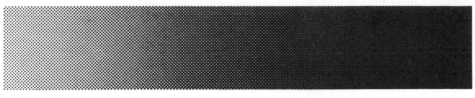

Inter-relationships

All the design principles described previously can be inter-related in many ways to produce effects such as movement or stillness, or even coldness or warmth. For example, a smooth bob hairstyle may be stiffly sprayed with hairspray to look still, whereas a long, bouncy curly hairstyle will have lots of movement. In a similar way ashen or blue-based hair colours have a cold appearance (cool white blondes) and redheads appear warm (fiery redheads).

DESIGNING A HAIRSTYLE FOR THE CLIENT

Body build and height

Hairstyles should not only make the most of facial features, but they must balance the client's body build and height.

SMALL Small clients can look overwhelmed by too much hair, or made to appear shorter from the back by wearing their hair too long.

MEDIUM Clients of medium build and medium height can take almost any hairstyle.

LARGE (OVERWEIGHT) Short, flat hairstyles can highlight bigness (turtle-like), whereas a style with some volume and length will create a balance.

TALL Tall clients suit simple, elegant hairstyles either long and full, or very short hair.

Head and neck shapes

HEAD SHAPES There are some head shapes where it is difficult to cut the hair into shorter styles because the head shapes are not quite perfect. Longer styles can be adapted by cutting and styling to minimize the faults, and create a more rounded shape.

Here are some examples showing different head shapes. The arrows explain where the hair should be shorter or closer to the head ↓ and where the hair should be longer or styled away from the head ↑.

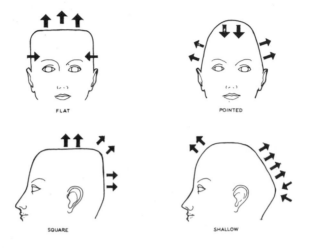

Head shapes

NECK SHAPES   Long and thin necks will be accentuated by short hairstyles and need longer hair around them. Short necks can be made to look longer by an upswept or flicked style.

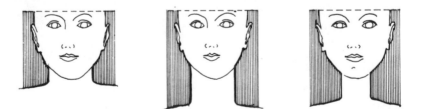

Hair characteristics

The type of hair (Caucasian, Negroid or Asian), the texture, the length, the volume the colour, the hairline (including any hair loss, the natural growth patterns and any previous treatments are fully described in Chapter 5).

ETHNIC GROUPS

European hair (Caucasian)   Caucasian hair may be straight, wavy or curly, of fine or coarse texture and of varying colours. It is, therefore, possible to style, cut, permanently wave, bleach and colour this hair easily.

Asian hair (Mongoloid)   This hair type is generally dark brown or black and often very straight. People often grow it long, have it cut and then sell it to wigmakers to be made into postiche. It may be cut easily, styled and permed but it is difficult to bleach to a light blonde in one application.

Negroid hair   This hair is generally very curly and usually dark brown or black. It may be styled and cut (see Chapters 7 and 8) easily, but perming and bleaching are more difficult procedures.

Hairlines

Facial hairlines can vary from client to client, and often the style must be adapted to suit them. Normal hairlines are easy to manage, but receding hairlines are often dressed forward to cover them. Very straight hairlines can accentuate round and square face shapes, and partings near the centre of the head are needed.

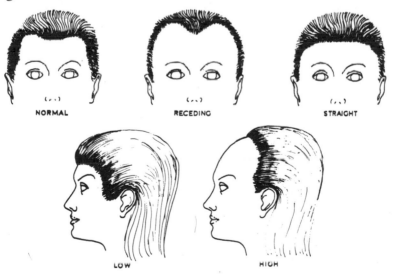

NORMAL   RECEDING   STRAIGHT

LOW   HIGH

Low hairlines are often dressed away from the face and high hairlines dressed towards the face to that they are not as noticeable.

Face shapes

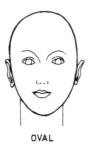

OVAL

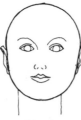

ROUND

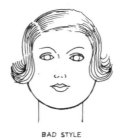

BAD STYLE

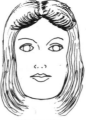

GOOD STYLE

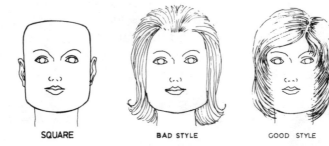

SQUARE   BAD STYLE   GOOD STYLE

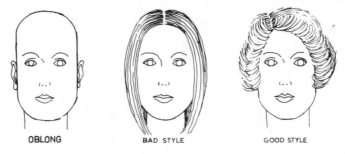

OBLONG   BAD STYLE   GOOD STYLE

OVAL   An oval face shape is the ideal and suits any hairstyle. Diamond and heart shapes are also good to work with.

SQUARE   Square shaped faces need high rounded dressings with wisps to soften them and give the illusion of appearing oval.

ROUND   Round faces need height which tends to reduce the width of the face. A straight centre parting will also reduce the width (page 252).

OBLONG   Long faces can be made to appear shorter and wider by being cut shorter and dressed around the sides of the face.

The bone structure of the face

THE BONES OF THE HEAD   The head is almost entirely made up of bones which protect the brain and delicate sense organs such as the eyes, ears, etc. In fact there are twenty-two bones which make up the skull, but all except the lower jaw (mandible) are rigidly fused together. The skull can be divided into two main areas, the face and the cranium.

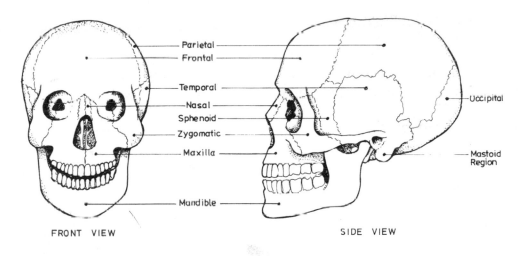

FRONT VIEW   SIDE VIEW

The main bones of the face are the jaw bones and cheek bones/ zygomatic bones. The eight bones of the cranium protect the brain.

THE MUSCLES OF THE HEAD   The muscles of the head lie between the skin and bones and form the flesh. As you will see from the diagram overleaf, there are many individual muscles which serve this area of the body, but all fulfil one or more of three functions:

1 **Facial expression** – most of the muscles of the face are involved in the formation of facial expression. A wide variety of facial expressions is possible, e.g. happy, surprised, angry, content, sad

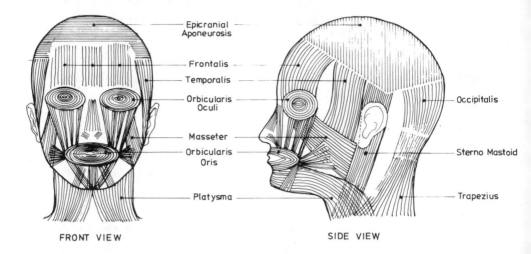

FRONT VIEW   SIDE VIEW

etc. Our facial expressions form a very important part of our non-verbal communications.

2 **Chewing (mastication)** – the masseter and the temporalis are the muscles most involved in chewing.
3 **Movement of head** – the sternomastoid and trapezius muscles are responsible for head movements.

Faces in profile

The design line of the hairstyle when viewed from the side can highlight the following features.

EYEBROWS   Short fringes or hair taken away from the face will highlight the eyebrows and may not always suit clients with bushy eyebrows.

If clients are considering changing their hair colour, than the natural colour of their eyebrows may not always match. Eyebrow tinting or bleaching is best carried out by a qualified beautician.

EYES   The choice of hair colour is again important to relate to the colour of the client's eyes, for example bleached hair suits clients with blue, grey or green eyes more than those with brown eyes.

MOUTHS   Large and full mouths are again accentuated by hair taken away from the face, which draws attention to them.

NOSES Large noses are accentuated by hair drawn back from the face, whereas a forward dressing will help to minimize them.

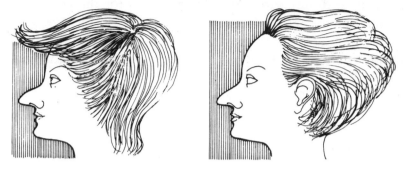

EARS Generally large ears, or even large lobes, are highlighted by hair either cut short or dressed away from the face.

Some clients have ears that are uneven, so never balance a haircut by the level of the ears!

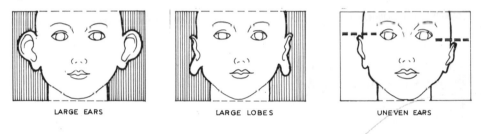

| LARGE EARS | LARGE LOBES | UNEVEN EARS |

Age

Styling to suit a client's age is not only relevant to cutting and styling (see Chapters 7 and 8), but also to her/his complexion, skin colour (see chapter 11) and make-up (see Chapter 3) are necessary considerations.

The client's life-style and financial considerations are equally important when choosing a style.

THE APPLICATION OF DESIGN PRINCIPLES

To apply the knowledge in this chapter you will need a sketchbook and pencil to try out the designs on paper before using the ideas on your client.

Discuss your ideas with the client and use a questionnaire to help you to remember both the questions to ask and the answers given.

An example of a questionnaire follows on the next page.

If you feel that drawing is not your strong point, then use examples of styles cut out from newspapers and magazines (do not use ones from newspapers and magazines kept in the salon for the clients to read), and then make your selection. You may also find examples of complete 'total looks' to interest your client, and if you have access to wigs, then clients may wish to try them to see instant changes!

Questionnaire for designing a suitable hairstyle

Client name:
Stylist name:
Client lifestyle and dress:
Approximate client age:
Financial considerations:
Client body build/height:
Head shape:
Neck shape:
Profile:
Hair characteristics (including ethnic origins):
Hairline:
Line of hairstyle – front view:
Line of hairstyle – side view:
Line of hairstyle – back view:
Partings (if applicable):
Volume of style:
Shape of style:
Balance of style:
Texture of style:
Haircolour (tone and depth, see Chapters 11, 12 and 13):
Face shape:
Special notes regarding eyebrows, eye colour, nose, mouth,
    ears, skin colour and make-up:
Client preferences:

MULTIPLE CHOICE QUESTIONS

1 A client with a full round face would be advised to adopt a style that adds:
(a) to the roundness of the face
(b) height and tends to reduce width of face
(c) width but not height of the face
(d) equal height and width to the face

2 A client who wishes to offset a long neck would be a advised to adopt style that is:
(a) across the nape
(b) V-shaped in the nape
(c) above the nape
(d) below the nape

3 A side parting will appear to:
(a) emphasize the nose
(b) highlight the cheek bones
(c) broaden the head
(d) darken sallow colours

4 Roughened cuticle scales may make the hair appear:
(a) dull   (c) dark
(b) shiny   (d) light

5 Harmonious colours are:
(a) secondary colours
(b) those which produce white when mixed
(c) opposite each other on the colour circle
(d) close together on the colour circle

6 Which of the following will help to balance a square face?
(a) soft rounded movements
(b) angular styles
(c) short tapered hair
(d) central parting

7 Which style would help to offset a long face?
(a) fringe and extra height
(b) long shoulder length hair with central parting
(c) fringe and side width
(d) very short hair with no fringe

8 During styling when only the roots are backcombed it is for:
(a) body   (c) volume
(b) lift   (d) fine hair

15

DESIGN STUDIES

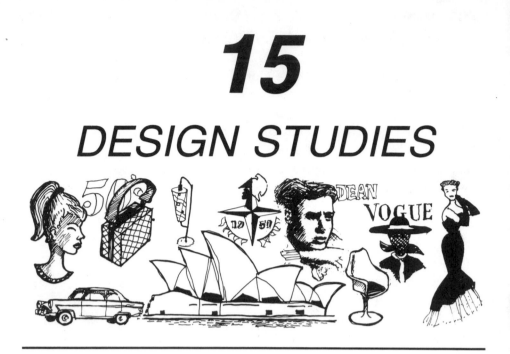

Once you have gained an understanding of the principles of design and its relevance to the practical aspects of hairdressing, then you may wish to continue a stage further through design studies.

You may have developed an interest in a fashion 'total look' and wish to produce your own style book, or a fashion show to promote your salon. 'Total looks' are also based on history from Egyptian to 1970's styles; which are often taken as themes in hairdressing shows and seminars.

If you wish to work in the theatre, the film or TV industry; or to dress wigs for life-size models in museums or shop-displays, then a historical knowledge is essential.

The design of the salon is also very important, not only from the practical sense of being able to move yourself and your client around the salon easily and safely, but for creating the right atmosphere. Colours, patterns, fabrics, displays, lighting, music and graphic design (i.e. lettering, signs, logos) contribute to make either a very attractive or a very unattractive salon.

TOTAL LOOKS

The relationship between hair design, fashion and make-up is often known as a 'total look'. A 'style' can run through many periods in art, whereas fashion is a reflection of that style. If design principles are ignored then the 'total look' will be poor and unco-ordinated. Make-up, accessories and clothes (see Chapter 3), skin tone and complexion (see Chapter 11) must all relate to the hairstyle. Many clients perceive 'total looks' through magazines and newspapers and this is where your own personalized style book is useful.

Style books

Manufacturers and publishers produce ready made style books but if you produce your own book you can highlight your special interests. You may be excited by new hair colours or permanent waves, or new fashionable haircuts, and by showing your style book to the client your enthusiasm will be seen more clearly.

Good presentation is vital. The book must be properly bound and made of a hardwearing material (such as plastic). The front cover should be illustrated with your salon name, or logo, and your name. Inside the book should be a brief introduction, followed by illustrations. These may be made by you, or cut out from magazines and attached to the sheets inside. The sheets should be protected from wet hands by acrylic, or use acrylic folder inserts which enable the illustrations to be slotted inside, and regularly changed. If clients see that you are interested in them as individuals, then you are more assured of repeated custom.

Style books can be used to illustrate everyday styles (see Chapters 7 and 8), or to promote hairstyles for special occasions.

HAIRSTYLES FOR SPECIAL OCCASIONS

Clients may ask for a suitable hairstyle for a special occasion such as a wedding, a dinner dance or a sophisticated theatre or opera visit. In such a case you will have to combine your knowledge of design principles with designing a new hairstyle.

These styles are generally more elaborate than everyday ones and may be decorated with ribbons, artificial flowers or hair ornaments. If the client has short hair then extra length or volume may be needed. This can be achieved by the use of postiche (added hair) or hair extensions.

Postiche

Hairpieces are attached by hairgrips and pins, and secured to a flat barrel curl (made from the clients own, dry, hair) which is held in place with hairgrips. Once the postiche is securely attached, then it may be dressed into a variety of styles.

Hairpieces can be made from either real hair or synthetic fibres (which look and feel very similar), and therefore may be different to dress out. Real hair has a cuticle scale and may be backcombed easily, but synthetic fibres have no cuticle scale and are sometimes difficult to backcomb. Real hair is **hygroscopic** and absorbs water which enables it to be set and curled with heated styling aids. Synthetic fibres are pre-curled, cannot be set, and will melt if heated styling aids are used.

To test if the hairpiece is real or synthetic, cut off a small strand, tie it with cotton, place in a safe container (such as a china saucer) and check that no inflammable materials are nearby. Carefully set light to it. If it crumbles and singes then it is real hair, but if it melts into a solid shape then it is made of synthetic fibre.

Long hair styles

Long hair may be curled by setting, blow drying or using heated styling aids to produce more volume, or it may be put up into smooth dressings. Sometimes stylists combine the two techniques by pulling the hair up, then allowing it to fall into a cascade of curls, ringlets or crimped hair. There are two simple upswept hairstyles, the French Pleat and the Chignon.

FRENCH PLEAT This is where the back of the hair is dressed smoothly across from behind the ears towards the.centre and twisted into a pleat or roll.

The front of the hair may be combed smoothly into it or styled in a variety of ways to suit the face shape (see Chapter 14).

CHIGNONS Chignons are often dressed in the back area of the head and may be twisted to form a knot or roll, or plaited and secured with hairgrips and pins.

TWISTS AND PLAITS If the hair is to be twisted or plaited, it must be divided into equal amounts and brushed or combed smoothly first. Here are some simple diagrams to help you practice:

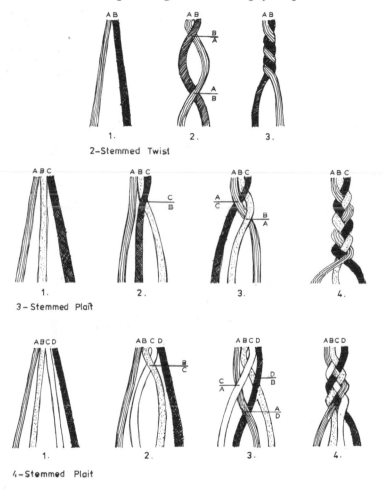

2–Stemmed Twist

3 – Stemmed Plait

4–Stemmed Plait

These twists and plaits are secured with special elasticated bands.

All long hair dressings should be smooth (without untidy back-combing) and hairgrips and pins must be hidden.

Hair extensions

Lengths of false hair, normally made from acrylic fibre, can be attached to the client's own hair by using a special technique. This looks good on layered, tapered or razored Caucasian hair or even better on Negroid hair. Extensions are best used around the back of the head where the hair is naturally thicker, or placed behind the front hairline so that they cannot easily be seen.

Acrylic hair extensions are light to wear, and although they cannot be brushed or combed, they can be carefully shampooed. As the client's hair starts to grow, they will gradually loosen and need to be replaced every few months. They cannot be tinted, bleached or permed as they are not hygroscopic, but they can be dressed in any of the variety of long hair dressings previously described.

Hair extensions are attached to the client's hair by taking small square sections divided into two (see Diagram 1). A suitable length and colour of acrylic hair can then be selected. The technique then requires the skills of two hairdressers. Each hairdresser holds two strands of hair in each hand. The two strands of the client's hair are held by one hairdresser, as the other inserts the acrylic hair folded in half (see Diagram 2). The first hairdresser then crosses the client's hair over the acrylic hair. The second hairdresser then crosses the acrylic hair over the client's hair (see Diagram 3).

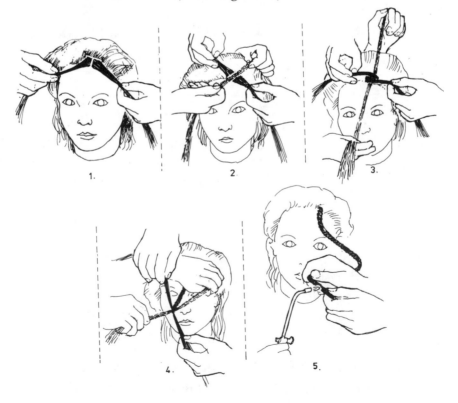

This is continued until the client's hair disappears inside the braid (see Diagram 4). The hairdressers must then seal the acrylic hair with heat to make it secure (see Diagram 5). The remaining hair may be left free, or twisted, braided and pleated.

Hair extensions are removed by twisting to break this seal, and then they may be unravelled.

FASHION SHOWS AND SEMINARS

Hairdressers work in a fashion industry and often wish to expres their own, or their salon's individual style.

Fashion shows to promote individual or group salons to the public, or hairdressing seminars to promote individual or group salons to other hairdressers, are a regular part of hairdressing life.

To produce a fashion show, expert advice is needed from professional people. These professionals will advise on stage lighting, music, choice of compere, rehearsals (timing is crucial), and the choice of models.

Shows are often 'themed' for example:

COLOUR THEMES The models' clothes may be colour co-ordinated. Black and white or neutrals are the easiest to use.

TIMES OF THE DAY Some of the models may wear day clothes whilst others may be in evening dress, with matching hairstyles.

SPECIAL OCCASIONS Wedding clothes, beach wear and sports-wear, all need suitable hairstyles specifically for that occasion.

ERAS Egyptian, Roman, Medieval, Elizabethan, the French Baroque, Victorian, Edwardian styles, or reflections of the 1920s, 1930s, 1940s, 1950s, 1960s and 1970s are often used.

ETHNIC THEMES These include African, Russian, South American or Oriental looks.

ORGANIZED GROUPS Military looks or American baseball teams are useful to show variations on one theme.

FANTASY LOOKS Creatures such as butterflies, snakes, birds and animals may be used as a basic theme for both colour and style.

CURRENT THEMES These may reflect current TV or radio shows, news items, (such as Royal Weddings), current music bands or vocalists or new films or theatre productions.

A HISTORICAL SURVEY OF STYLES

Egyptians

The first elaborate hairstyles were worn by the Egyptians, who shaved their heads because of the heat, and wore decorative wigs. These were often made from human hair and coloured with different natural hair dyes, such as Henna.

Egyptians often wore elaborate head-dresses and heavy eye make-up.

The architectural pyramids of Egypt were reflected in the strong geometric shapes of the hairstyles, make-up and clothes. Egyptian hieroglyphics were the written words of the time and can be seen in their design patterns.

Greeks

Greeks mostly wore their hair short and softly curled, but longer hair was worn up and tied with ribbons or braids.

In the same way that Greek philosophers tried to bring ideas together, their logical architecture (i.e. pillars held together by level beams) is reflected in the way that hair was loosely tied together.

Flowing robes were worn because of the heat, and were fastened loosely around the body.

The decoration at the top of the pillars in the temples can be seen on both the exteriors and interiors of many buildings.

Greek key patterns are often seen on borders around rooms and also around the edges of fabric.

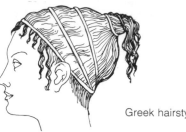

Greek hairstyle

Romans

During Roman times hair started to become more elaborate, often put up and with braids or curls.

At one time prostitutes were required either to dye their hair yellow or to wear yellow wigs, but later yellow hair became fashionable for everyone.

Roman and Greek hairstyles were quite similar and so too were their clothes, the Roman toga being the most famous.

Architecture and decoration became more elaborate, but still based on geometry. The Pantheon in Rome is a good example of this.

Medieval

After the Dark Ages came the medieval times and from the 12th century to the 14th century the church grew in power, the people becoming more orderly and civilized. Hair, if not completely covered by head-dresses and veils was plaited, braided or coiled over the ears (and sometimes padded with false hair, cotton, or wool). Occasionally front hairlines were shaved or the hair was plucked away.

Gothic architecture of the time reflected the influence of the church with high vaulted ceilings and flying buttresses.

Renaissance

The 15th century in Italy saw a great revival of the arts known as the High Renaissance, which produced remarkable artists such as Leonardo da Vinci, Michelangelo, Raphael and Botticelli. They sometimes painted portraits of powerful families such as the Borgias and the Medicis, and the hairstyles were very decorative.

In England head-dresses were becoming more elaborate, as the arts there also started to flourish.

Italian Renaissance architecture (the most famous Italian architect of the time being Palladio), reflected both Greek and Roman architecture and can still be seen today throughout Italy.

The Tudors and Elizabethans

The influence of the Italian Renaissance began to be seen in England in the 16th century, and short hair became fashionable.

Both men and women began to wear ruffs around their necks and clothes became more elaborately decorated. Men began to grow beards which were often neatly trimmed, whilst women wore their hair in a similar style to that of Queen Elizabeth I (even dying or powdering their hair the same colour).

Titian was a famous Italian painter of that time, and we still refer to 'Titian red hair'.

In Tudor and Elizabethan times the influence of architecture was beginning to be seen in people's homes as well as churches and palaces. It is still possible to see the carved wood panels and windows decorated with heraldic symbols in buildings such as Hampton Court Palace.

The Jacobeans

During the reign of Charles II in the 17th century, the Royalists or Cavaliers wore very elaborate hair styles. Men wore full-bottomed black wigs which were a mass of tumbling ringlets and often made from horse hair.

Women also wore ringlets, curls and hair ornaments (such as pearls) in their hair, but the later influence of Oliver Cromwell produced the Puritan style which was smoother and simpler.

French Baroque

During the reign of Louis XIV (the Sun King) of France in the 18th century, not only did hairstyles become very exaggerated, but also the palaces became heavily decorated and ornamented. Versailles Palace (outside Paris) is a good example of this, containing vast flights of steps, many statues and elaborate fountains. 'Trompe L'Oeil', which is where a wall painting gives the illusion of either the interior or the exterior of the building being continued, was often used in the Baroque period.

During this period, (just before the French Revolution) many wigs were used and they were often powdered and dusted with either wheat flour or sifted starch mixed with plaster-of-Paris. 'Macaroni' wigs (of Italian influence) were worn by men, and one popular style for women was brushed back from the face and called the 'Pompadour' style. Women's wigs were heavily ornamented with lace, ribbons, artificial flowers and pearls.

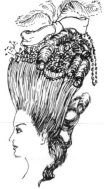

Pompadour style

People also powdered their faces and wore small black patches in the shape of beauty spots or crescents.

English hairdressing and make-up was influenced by the French Baroque style, and produced a similar style called Rococco.

The formality of Georgian architecture was seen in both towns (e.g. London's squares) and country.

Interiors began to be decorated with wallpapers, silks and satin hangings and painted porcelain china became very popular.

Regency

At the beginning of the 19th century, a small group of men called 'dandies' including George (Beau) Brummell, influenced both dress and hair fashions. Men no longer wore wigs, but kept their hair short at the back (because they wore high collars), with curls, fringes and waves at the front. Long side-burns and whiskers also became fashionable.

At this time women often wore their hair piled up in a chignon or topknot with curls at the side. Hair was also worn in the Greek style and there was a revival of loose dresses, tied under the bust. Classical architecture reflecting the styles of ancient Greece and Rome, became popular and was reflected in the beautiful Regency buildings, (such as those in the City of Bath) which can still be seen today.

More interest grew in landscaping too, (as can be seen at places such as Stourhead in Wiltshire) and the countryside was depicted by painters such as Constable.

Victorian

During the last part of the 19th century when Queen Victoria reigned, men's hairstyles remained similar, but whiskers became neater and heavy 'cavalry' moustaches became popular. Women's hair was still upswept in the middle 1850s, but the chignons were worn low in the back of the neck, often held in place with ivory and tortoiseshell combs and hairpins, and ringlets were popular.

By the 1870s hair became softer with longer curls worn at the back and red hair was fashionable. This was because of the influence of the Pre-Raphaelite painters such as Rosetti. However, not everyone had curly hair, and in 1888 Marcel invented the first heated waving irons which produced both waves and curls.

Victorian interiors were over ornamented and decorated, and rooms were full of furniture, heavy curtains, wall pictures and patterned wallpapers. The 'Arts and Crafts' movement influenced wallpaper and fabric design. This became known as 'Art Nouveau'.

Architecture was also heavily decorated and examples of this are the Houses of Parliament and the Victoria and Albert museum.

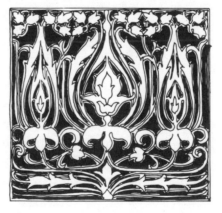

Edwardian

At the beginning of this century women's hair was still worn curly but swept upwards.

There was a short fashion for blond hair reflecting the popularity of Lily Langtry (a famous actress) but then auburn hair became popular again and Henna was used to create this effect. By 1910 cosmetics were first sold openly, and became respectable. They had previously only been used by prostitutes.

During Edwardian times people travelled more, ornaments from the British Empire were often seen around the rooms. Architecture reflected modern art, and flat roofed buildings, such as those designed by Frank Lloyd Wright were being built.

The 1920s

During the First World War (1914–1918) women who worked in factories found their long hair both a nuisance and dangerous and so began to have their hair cut shorter. The influence of Emily Pankhurst, who fought for women's rights, led to clothes becoming looser (dresses appeared without tight waistlines) and new hairstyles. The 'bob' was introduced, gradually becoming shorter and called a 'semi-shingle', and developing into the 'Eton Crop'.

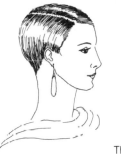

The Eton Crop

Women's make-up also became stronger. Eyebrows were plucked to a fine line and mouths were painted strong red colours.

Men's hair developed in a similar fashion – soldiers in the war had to have their hair cut short because of the spread of head infestations (such as head lice) while they were living so closely together in the trenches. The shingled style continued into the 1950s and is still popular with mature clients today.

As technology advanced in the 20th century, it became possible to build tall skyscraper buildings such as those in Manhatten, New York, but it was still fashionable to decorate them at that time. The Chrysler building is the best known example of this.

The 1930s

The modernist movement, which reflected angular patterns and shapes, was seen in art and architecture at this time.

Many contemporary buildings were similar to those designed at the Bauhaus, an art school in Germany founded by Walter Gropius.

Cinemas and interiors began to change from being heavily decorated to a more functional style called Art Deco.

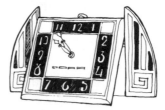

Art Deco style

At this time the film industry began to develop, using both colour and sound, and people began visiting the cinema regularly. Women could see actresses with new hairstyles and changes became more frequent.

Hair became curlier as permanent wave machines became common in salons, and although hair was still flat, it was softer at the sides.

The 1940s

The Second World War (1939–1945) had a strong influence on women's hairstyles. Many women again worked in the factories (as the men were fighting in the war) and their longer hair was curled under (to keep it safe from machines) in a 'Page Boy' hairstyle.

After the war, men began to wear their hair longer on top, and the fashion for this began to develop.

The 1950s

The post war years were times of hardship with food and furniture rationing, but when the economy started to improve so did the interest in hairdressing. Most women set their hair in rollers to achieve curls and lift, and the 'Bubble Cut' was very popular.

The 'Italian Boy' style which was taken back off the face was popularized by Queen Elizabeth II, and is still in demand today. Women began to wear more make-up, and for the first time the younger generation developed their own style of clothes, for example the 'Teddy Boy' suit.

Architecture and interiors became more decorated. Flats were brightened on the outside by chequerboard patterns of varied colours, and houseplants, both real and plastic, featured in most homes.

The 1960s

This era saw one of the most dramatic changes in hair and clothes fashiones. Music bands such as the Beatles and the Rolling Stones and the English clothes designer Mary Quant had a strong impact. The 'mini-skirt' was introduced, and girls wore pale make-up, pale lipstick and heavy eye-make-up (false eyelashes were very popular).

Hairdressing styles changed from becoming more and more backcombed ('Beehives') to being blow dried instead of set. The hairdresser Vidal Sassoon introduced the 'precision cut', and bobs of varying lengths became very popular.

Asymetrical hairstyles (see Chapter 14, page 256), and geometric cuts developed alongside the fashion for 'Op Art' which created optical illusions; this was a direct influence from the Bauhaus movement in the 1930s. Geometric patterned prints featured on clothing and accessories such as earrings, necklaces, bags, gloves and shoes.

Architecture also became exaggerated and many high-rise flats were built during this era.

The 1970s

The 1970s saw a move away from angular forms and fashion became more romantic. Less tailored, floral printed clothes and accessories gave rise to the term 'flower power' and many young people grew their hair long and unkempt ('hippies'). Body make-up became popular, and for a brief time even flowers were painted on the skin.

Towards the end of this decade came another fashion change – the 'Punk' look, e.g. Sid Vicious, where clothes were worn shredded and tattered, and held together with safety pins. Make-up became very strong and exaggerated as did the hairstyles. Bright coloured, spiked hair was very fashionable, often completely shaved away at the sides (a 'Mohican' look).

During this decade interiors became more 'earthy' (brown was the most popular colour) and natural textured fabrics were widely used with the 'back to nature' revival. People started to move away from high-rise flats and live in small groups of houses. This was called 'Community Architecture'. Art posters became widely available and many Pre-Raphaelite, romantic illustrations decorated the walls.

Historical references for further research

Victoria and Albert Museum – Cromwell Road, London SW7
British Museum – Gt. Russell Street, London WC1
National Portrait Gallery – Trafalgar Square, London WC2
British Film Institute – Publications, 81 Dean Street, London W1V 6AA
Historical Hair Museum – The Wella Museum
            Berliaer, Allee 65,
            61 Darmstadt,
            West Germany.

SALON DESIGN

Exteriors

Clients unless personally recommended to the salon, will have been attracted by the outside from a distance, and by the reception area if they are walking past.

The outside should blend with the buildings surrounding it, for example a 'high tech' modern salon would be out of place in a Georgian conservation area. The salon name should suit the type of salon, for example during the 1950s French 'chic' was popular (Paris was then the centre of the fashion world), and salons may have been called 'Maison Coiffure'!

The style of lettering is also important and changes with fashion.

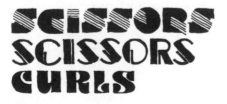

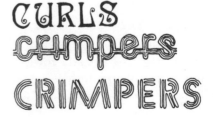

Sometimes the salon name is the logo, whereas the logo may be designed around or next to the name.

Another example of a common symbol used is the red and white barber's pole.

Names are often either on brightly coloured backgrounds or lit up from above or below to make them stand out.

Most salons have a glass fascia (or frontage) so that clients can see inside, and either exterior or interior sun blinds may be used. Interior blinds can be either horizontal or vertical, fine or wide Venetian, Festoon or Roman, with fabrics to match the salon colours. Curtains are occasionally used, depending on the fashion of the salon.

WINDOW DISPLAYS The current open-plan salon style often needs a less cluttered display. Displays can be two dimensional, i.e. posters, photographs or price lists, or three dimensional, i.e. products, hairdressing equipment or sculptures (display heads).

All displays, whether they are in the front window or inside the salon must be well presented, not untidy, badly positioned, dusty, or badly lit.

Temporary displays, such as salon promotions (special offers), should be changed regularly, and permanent displays such as jewellery and hair ornaments must be regularly checked, because sunlight will fade the packaging.

When you are designing a display always look at the background behind it, for instance earrings against a small patterned print will disappear!

Life-size sculptured heads are easy to make with modelling clay, and polystyrene heads are inexpensive to decorate with paint, wool, string, wire, card or foil. Remember to look at the background as silhouettes can be confusing!

Figure ground shapes

The Reception Area

The reception desk and chair should be easily visible from the door, but if the salon is on an upper floor, with a staircase leading to it, then there must be clear directional signs.

Signs can be professionally made with plastic or metal backing or hand made by printing, Letrasetting, or by using felt tip pens. The lettering must be clear (and not mis-spelt), level and clean (not smudged). Signs are often covered with a thin seal of self-clinging acetate to keep them clean, and must be positioned so that they are visible when viewed from different positions.

Coat cupboards and toilets often have signs or symbols, so decide which is most suitable for your salon style.

Posters are often displayed in reception areas, sometimes to promote retail products or sales promotions (such as reduced price permanent waves), and can be either made professionally or by hand. If so, the same lettering rules apply as for signwriting, but illustrations may be better done by professionals. Most manufacturers regularly produce show cards, which are well photographed, but make sure they are clearly positioned and securely in place.

Price lists may be displayed either in the window or near the reception area, and are usually professionally made. The written words and the numerals may be either slotted into place or stuck on to a magnetic board, so that they can be changed easily.

Flower displays and indoor plants often feature at the reception area and it is important that they are well cared for and watered regularly. Attractive silk imitation plants are now readily available.

If magazine and style books are kept at the reception area then they should be up-to-date and neatly arranged.

The seating at reception is usually more comfortable (to allow clients to relax) than the rest of the salon furniture, which must be more hardwearing.

In the same way the lighting should be softer (different lampshades are sometimes used) to help the clients relax. The only strong lighting should be to highlight retail displays.

Interiors

The planning of the salon is the most important decision to make. This means where the basins, dressing tables, chairs and trolleys are positioned, where the entrances and exits are and whether staff and clients can easily and safely move around the salon. It is always wise to seek professional advice from an architect to make sure that it is planned correctly, and that the services such as the water supplies and electricity work properly. A general guide to the amount of work space needed is approximately 1 sq. metre per operator (stylist).

The style of the interior generally matches that of the exterior. It may be Victorian or Art Nouveau, Modern (1920s), Art Deco (1930s), 1950s, 'Op' Art (1960s) or country style (1970s). The 'high tech' look of the 1980s exposes all the internal machinery (water pipes, electricity cables, ventilation ducts) so that it is all visible. A good example of this is the Pompidou centre in Paris or the Lloyds Building in London.

The fabrics and textures of the wallpapers, curtains or blinds and seating materials should blend together, and also complement the flooring. Salon floors must be very hardwearing and non-slip to withstand both chemical spillages and high heeled stiletto shoes.

The colours used in salons should reflect the style used. For instance country styles often use soft browns, beiges, greens, blues, pinks and yellows, whereas modern, high-tech, salons are often black, white, grey and chrome. Colours must harmonize (see Chapter 14) if it is a relaxing salon, but a 'punk' salon should be reflected by the use of brighter colours.

Some salons have specialist areas for tinting and perming where the colours and lighting are crucial to the finished hair colour result (see page 214) and others have specialist areas for children. Young children may be nervous and frightened when they first visit the salon, so the atmosphere of their specialist area should make them feel more relaxed. If there is enough space (for instance in large department stores), then sometimes chairs are adapted to look like toy cars or animals to make the visit more enjoyable.

SALON PROMOTIONS

New salons often need to promote themselves to become more widely known, and this may be done through advertising in newspapers and magazines. The wording, lettering and visual illustrations are all equally important. Psychologically, people remember visual illustrations more than written words, so salon logos are vital.

Posters, brochures, fashion show tickets, carrier bags and T-shirts will all help to promote the salon if they are well designed.

Many manufacturers produce specialist products to retail such as shampoos, conditioners and hairsprays which come complete with stands, but salons can buy the unlabelled products and use their own logo for further promotion (see page 161).

In the same way that manufacturers' showcards can be hung on the walls, it is possible to display and frame your own artwork or enlarged photographed hairstyles for display. It is important that they are well presented and well lit, and that the background does not detract from them.

DESIGNING FOR 'YOUR' SALON

You may decide that your salon would benefit from some two-dimensional artwork; either signs, posters, a new logo (for packaging letterheads or salon promotions), personalized fabric design (for blinds) or even three-dimensional work such as display heads. Start by doing some research.

Firstly, think about the style of your salon, then the colours and the textures around you. If there are some bare walls, the window display needs more interest or the salon needs a new image then start to work out your ideas on paper, and organize them into order.

Tools and equipment for designing

PENCILS   B pencils, such as 2B, 4B and 5B are soft leads and good for shading. You can buy special fixative to prevent sketches from smudging.

PASTELS   These are coloured pencils which can be mixed with water to create a 'wash' effect.

FELT-TIP PENS   These are often used for signwriting and are available in various thicknesses. It is possible to shade drawings with felt tip pens by using the 'Dot' technique. If you space dots closely together you can create dark tones, and if you space the same dots further apart you can create light tones.

PEN AND INK   Pens and inks may be used to draw fine or thick lines or for ink washes (look at some Japanese prints).

BRUSHES   To develop your painting techniques, you will need a very fine, a medium and a thick paintbrush made of nylon (mock sable).

PAPER   Sketch books should contain good quality cartridge paper of A3 or A4 size.

STENCILS   To create a professional, clean artline, ready made stencils can be purchased, but it is possible to make your own.

Commercial techniques

If you wish to copy a drawing or a photograph (make sure it is not copyright), then photocopiers are are readily available. It is possible to enlarge and reduce on paper and on acetate sheets (for overhead projector use) by using photocopying facilities.

COLLAGE   This is when materials such as string or wool are used to simplify shapes (especially hair) and attached (by glue) to a background. Magazine cut outs can be used in the same way (a good example of collage is Peter Blake's work). Photomontage is where separate photographs are blended together to form one picture.

FABRIC   It is possible to stencil onto fabric, as it is possible to stencil colours and patterns on to hair, but precise patterns are difficult to achieve. To repeat a pattern, lino cuts may be used, and this is how the first wallpaper patterns were achieved.

Tie-dyeing and Batik (which uses wax) give an abstract sometimes crackled effect but the colours must be carefully chosen beforehand (see Chapter 14, page 256).

Colours may be blended by using those close together on the colour wheel, e.g. reds, yellows, and oranges or perhaps blues and greens (analonous harmony). In the same way lighter and darker shades of the same colour tone e.g. pale red, red, and dark red may be combined (monochromatic harmony). Even colours directly opposite on the colour wheel, e.g. red and green will harmonize (complementary harmony) if they are the same depth of colour.

Fabric designs may be made into garments or framed if they have been card mounted, or even used for roller blinds (roller blind kits are readily available).

THREE-DIMENSIONAL WORK   This can be free-standing as with pieces of sculpture (display heads) or relief, which is sculpture fixed to a backing.

It is expensive to make a life-size display head from modelling clay, but polystyrene head forms are available from hairdressing wholesale houses. These can be decorated with wool, feathers, beads, card, paper and sequins or even padded out to extend the head shape.

Remember to stand back to look at the outline shape whilst working with three-dimensional sculpture in the same way as you would create a hairstyle.

FINAL NOTE

To be a good, competent hairdresser you not only need to be literate and numerate but you will need to develop some of the skills of a painter, sculptor, chemist, dermatologist and psychologist. You will also need lots of stamina!

Remember to use what you have learned. Clients often visit salons because they are lacking in self-confidence and need a new image. Think about design principles, lifestyles and financial considerations and suggest a suitable service for that individual client.

Clients today are well informed and do have a choice of salons – make sure it's yours!

ANSWERS

Chapter 2

1 (d)	2 (c)	3 (c)
4 (b)	5 (c)	6 (a)
7 (b)	8 (a)	9 (c)
10 (a)	11 (d)	12 (b)
13 (c)	14 (d)	15 (b)

Chapter 3

1 (a)	2 (d)	3 (c)
4 (a)	5 (c)	6 (b)
7 (d)	8 (a)	

Chapter 4

1 (c)	**2** (d)	**3** (b)
4 (a)	**5** (b)	**6** (d)
7 (c)	**8** (b)	**9** (a)
10 (a)	**11** (d)	

Chapter 5

1 (d)	**2** (a)	**3** (d)
4 (a)	**5** (b)	**6** (d)
7 (a)	**8** (b)	**9** (a)
10 (a)	**11** (c)	**12** (a)
13 (d)	**14** (a)	**15** (a)

Chapter 6

1 (d)	**2** (b)	**3** (a)
4 (b)	**5** (d)	**6** (a)
7 (a)	**8** (c)	**9** (b)
10 (c)	**11** (c)	**12** (a)
13 (c)	**14** (d)	**15** (b)

Chapter 7

1 (c)	**2** (a)	**3** (b)
4 (b)	**5** (a)	**6** (d)
7 (a)	**8** (b)	**9** (a)
10 (d)	**11** (d)	**12** (a)
13 (c)	**14** (a)	**15** (d)

Chapter 8

1 (a)	**2** (c)	**3** (a)
4 (a)	**5** (d)	**6** (d)
7 (c)	**8** (a)	**9** (d)
10 (b)		

Chapter 9

1 (d)	2 (a)	3 (b)
4 (a)	5 (b)	6 (c)
7 (d)	8 (a)	9 (b)
10 (d)	11 (c)	12 (a)
13 (b)	14 (d)	

Chapter 10

1 (b)	2 (b)	3 (d)
4 (c)	5 (c)	6 (b)
7 (a)	8 (c)	9 (a)
10 (d)	11 (c)	12 (a)
13 (d)	14 (b)	15 (d)

Chapter 11

1 (d)	2 (d)	3 (b)
4 (c)	5 (a)	6 (c)
7 (b)	8 (d)	9 (c)
10 (c)	11 (a)	12 (d)
13 (a)	14 (b)	

Chapter 12

1 (d)	2 (a)	3 (c)
4 (b)	5 (d)	6 (a)
7 (b)	8 (a)	9 (c)
10 (a)	11 (b)	12 (c)
13 (c)	14 (d)	

Chapter 13

1 (d)	2 (a)	3 (c)
4 (b)	5 (d)	6 (a)
7 (b)	8 (a)	

Chapter 14

1 (b)	2 (d)	3 (c)
4 (a)	5 (d)	6 (a)
7 (c)	8 (b)	

GLOSSARY/INDEX

Contact Dermatitis   Inflammation of the skin following contact with certain chemicals, allergic reaction 69

Contagious   The transfer of disease by direct contact 14

Contour Products   Make-up 32

Contra-indication   A factor which dictates that hairdressing services should *not* be carried out, e.g. infestation 66

Convection   Transfer of heat through liquids or gas by means of convection currents 56

Convex Mirrors   Outwardly curving mirrors 42

Copper Sulphate   A metal salt found in metallic dyes 211

Cortex   Middle layer of hair. Forms main bulk of hair 70

Cosmetics   31

Cow's Lick   Growth pattern of hair at the front hairline 132

Cream   An emulsion 52

Cream Bleach   226

Cream Tints   200

Crimping Irons   118

Croquinole   Winding hair on rollers from the points 105

Curly Hair   75

Current Electricity   Flow of electricity through a circuit 20

Customer Relations   58

Curling Tongs   For heat styling 116

Cuts   9

Cuticle   Outer layer of hair 70

Cut Throat Razor   137

Cutting Tools   133

Cutting the Hair   Ch. 8

Dandruff   (Pityriasis simplex) excess shedding of the skin on the scalp 68

Deionised Water   Water which has been treated to remove impurities 79

Density   Measurement involving volume and weight 54

Deodorants   Mask smells 30

Depth and Tone   Hair Colour chart 206

Dermatitis   Inflammation of skin 69

Dermis   Inner layer of skin 67

Design   Chapters 14 and 15

Designing a Hairstyle   251

Designing a salon   280–283

Detergency   79

Detergents   81

Diffused Light   Reflection of light by rough surface 74

Dilution   Of hydrogen peroxide 229

Direct Current   (Electricity) The electricity flows in one direction only 20